The Psychology of Panic

Edited by Robert W. Motta

Published in London, United Kingdom

The Psychology of Panic
http://dx.doi.org/10.5772/intechopen.102252
Edited by Robert W. Motta

Contributors
Olga Lainidi, Anthony Montgomery, Eva Tzioti, Panagiota Koutsimani, Maria Spiliou, Lin Wang, Yihao Liu, Seth Davin Norrholm, Behrooz Afshari, Bhupendra Singh Gurung, Robert W. Motta, Kaveh Moghaddam

First published in London, United Kingdom, 2023 by IntechOpen
IntechOpen is the global imprint of INTECHOPEN LIMITED, registered in England and Wales, registration number: 11086078, 5 Princes Gate Court, London, SW7 2QJ, United Kingdom

British Library Cataloguing-in-Publication Data
A catalogue record for this book is available from the British Library

Additional hard and PDF copies can be obtained from orders@intechopen.com

The Psychology of Panic
Edited by Robert W. Motta
p. cm.
Print ISBN 978-1-80356-647-4
Online ISBN 978-1-80356-648-1
eBook (PDF) ISBN 978-1-80356-649-8

Meet the editor

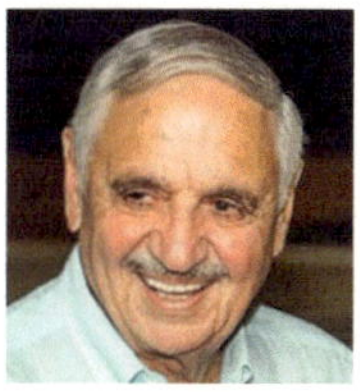

Robert W. Motta, Ph.D., ABPP, is a Professor Emeritus of Psychology and founder of the Child and Family Trauma Institute at Hofstra University, New York. There he served as the chairperson of the Psychology Department and founded an American Psychological Association (APA) accredited PsyD psychology doctoral program. He has published more than 100 scientific papers and book chapters as well as three books: *Alternative Therapies for PTSD The Science of Mind-Body Treatments*; *Altered: A Trauma and PTSD Casebook*; and *Suicide.* Dr. Motta is board certified in cognitive-behavioral psychology and behavior therapy. He is the former president of the School Division of the New York Psychological Association and is licensed as a clinical psychologist and certified as a school psychologist.

Contents

Preface

This book examines the psychological phenomenon of panic disorder. Specific examples are given involving cases that have been treated for the disorder with a variety of therapeutic interventions. These interventions include, but are not limited to, cognitive-behavioral psychotherapy, mindfulness meditation, exposure therapy, physical exercise, medications, immune system enhancers, and others. There is an exploration of both childhood and adult forms of panic that might take place in work environments. An effort is made to provide the reader with an understanding of panic disorder as a phenomenon that is distinct from more commonly seen anxiety attacks. Whereas anxiety may be experienced as an annoying and persistent discomfort, panic is a far more intense phenomenon. Panic attacks come on unexpectedly and afflict victims with an overwhelming sensation of dread and often a fear of complete annihilation. Panic is frequently associated with physiological sensations that are so extreme that the sufferer may feel that they are about to die. Once a panic attack is in progress there is little that can be done for the sufferer other than to provide them with support and encouragement and to simply be present for them and assure them that the attack will pass. In virtually all instances panic attacks are relatively brief episodes, although the book describes some rare cases in which panic can last for considerably longer time periods. Much about panic disorder remains unknown to this day, including why some are afflicted by it and some are not. This book is an effort to increase our understanding of panic disorder and how it can be managed.

Robert W. Motta
Psychology Department,
Hofstra University,
Hempstead, New York, USA

Section 1

Panic Disorder Perspectives

Chapter 1

Perspective Chapter: Panic Disorder – A Real-World Case Due to Covid

Robert W. Motta

Abstract

This chapter presents a "real-world" case of extreme panic disorder and details the treatments that were brought to bear in efforts to reduce the panic. Unlike most cases of panic which appear to arise unpredictably and from unknown causes and last for a short amount of time, this one was attributed to an underlying neurological condition and many of the extreme panic episodes persisted for full days. The condition producing this panic was autoimmune encephalitis which appears to have arisen because of a Covid infection. The eventual resolution of the panic disorder took almost 2 years of daily struggles and are detailed within the chapter.

Keywords: panic, Covid, autoimmune encephalitis, CBT, IVIG therapy, steroids, rituximab

1. Introduction

Many of the chapters in this book on the Psychology of Panic deal with important topics such as the etiologies of panic, its characteristics, its epidemiology, and interventions. What will be presented in this chapter is a real-world case of Jordan with whom I have been directly involved as a treating psychologist and who has experienced extreme and extended bouts of panic which appear to have resulted from Covid exposure and resulting neurological inflammation.

Before delving into the case, it is important to consider what a panic attack might be like on a personal level. The DSM-5 [1] provides specific criteria for defining panic and these specifics are addressed in more than one chapter in this book. But such analytic descriptions with their enumeration of a series of diagnostic criteria provide a somewhat antiseptic and emotionally detached view of a disorder that is difficult to identify with unless the reader has experienced panic attacks themselves. So let us try a different approach.

Imagine that you are driving home on a dark stormy night where the windswept rain is so intense that your car's windshield wipers, although on high, make the road ahead almost indistinguishable. You are on high alert and are driving slowly to avert any storm related difficulties and you can feel your heart beating because of the stress of driving through this intense storm. You come to a familiar railroad crossing and as you begin to approach it you both hear and feel your car's engine begin to run rough and stumble. Suddenly the engine dies and although your foot is off the brake, the car comes to a stop directly on the railroad tracks. Your fear level is now intensified. You are stuck on the tracks. Suddenly, you see brightly flashing red lights and ringing and realize that the railroad barrier arms are coming down in front of and behind your car and are a signal of an approaching train. You are trapped between the barriers and your car is sitting right in the middle of the tracks. A bright white light begins to appear out of the drenching rain, and you hear the horn of the train growing louder as it is rapidly approaching. You now are desperately trying to restart the car to move it either backward or forward to get off the tracks. You are gripped by a wild fear of impending annihilation by a locomotive that is now clearly in view and growing both louder and larger. You can feel the vibrations of this massive train as it literally shakes the tracks that you and your car are sitting on. You are about to be crushed and now your body tenses as you close your eyes knowing that in the next instant you and your car will be annihilated.

That feeling of being completely out of control and unable to affect your environment while also experiencing the extremely intense fear of annihilation is what a panic attack might feel like. The level of fear is so intense that all reason and problem solving become nonexistent. It is as if the thinking part of the brain has been shut down and an animal-like, reflexive, fleeing or freezing response takes hold. The term "fear" does not do justice to what a panic attack might feel like. It is a primal experience that is far beyond fear. It is often unimaginably intense and renders the suffer helpless and frantic.

According to the *Diagnostic and statistical Manual of Mental Disorders* [1] under normal circumstances panic attacks are relatively brief and can come on suddenly and unexpectedly. For example, one can be in a relaxed state or even emerging from sleep and suddenly experience a panic attack. In Jordan's case the panic attacks would often go on for hours and often consume a major part of the day. These extended episodes of panic are unusual and were later seen as originating from nervous system impairment due to Covid infection.

2. Case description

I had seen Jordan on and off for several years for a series of relatively minor issues that might be described as problems of living. He had self-doubts about his capabilities although he was both bright and well educated. As a 51-year-old he experienced bouts of depression, but these too were relatively mild and might be better described as episodes of melancholy. He also had a relatively low-level generalized anxiety disorder. He seemed unable to develop long term committed relationships despite having dated numerous women who he met on a variety of dating apps. Jordan was able to live on his own in New York City but often received financial support from his twin sister and his mother. At the time of his decent into panic, he was working as an adjunct professor teaching a variety of graduate and undergraduate psychology courses and three different universities.

Jordan's mother became infected with the Covid virus at age 75 and experienced a series of long-haul symptoms that lasted nearly a year. These included body pains, extreme fatigue, balance problems, memory difficulties and disorientation. The doctors who ultimately treated Jordan believed that although he likely caught Covid from his mother and he initially experienced only mild to minimal symptoms of Covid, as time progressed his symptoms slowly began to worsen. Their final diagnosis was that his Covid infection triggered autoimmune encephalitis whereby the immune system, in an overreaction to viral infection, began attacking the healthy tissue of Jordan's brain.

According to Younger [2], viruses can attack the body and produce a response the follows a specific sequence. The first stage of this sequence is the viral infection. This is then followed by an immune response and this response is followed by and manifests itself as an inflammatory process. Infection, immune response, and inflammation is referred to by Younger as "I-cubed" (p. 7). The immune system responds to the newly present virus as a pathogen that exists in the nervous system and attacks the nervous system to ward of the invader. Over time a neural cycle develops in which panic or pain become almost reflexive behavioral responses to invasion by the pathogen [3]. Treatment is often aimed at reducing the inflammation that was caused by the body's overactive immune response. Common outcomes of the inflammatory response are pain, depression, anxiety, fatigue, and attention problems. In Jordan's case his primary responses were extreme anxiety and panic, debilitating fatigue, and moderate depression.

3. Developmental course

Jordan reached out to me while he was still employed as an adjunct professor. Although popular and well regarded as a capable instructor, he reported that he was experiencing increasingly intense bouts of anxiety and that he was having difficulty getting through his day. Normally he was at ease and confident as an instructor, but he was now experiencing feelings of failure and simply getting himself into the classroom to teach was becoming increasing frightening and difficult. He felt that he could not present the material clearly and that students were noticing that his lectures were more and more disorganized. His normal easygoing demeanor was being replaced by an unhappy, ill at ease presence. Although he was able to see his classes through until the end of the semester, he knew that he would be unable to return. The anxiety he was experiencing made the thought of returning to the classroom a challenge that he was unable to meet.

Over time he began to become increasing anxious and feel threatened in situations that were normally soothing to him. For example, he enjoyed going to his gym which had a swimming pool. Swimming for Jordan was a stress reliever and a form of meditation. He was able to clear his mind of daily problems while swimming back and forth in the pool. All of this changed following his Covid infection. Eventually the thought of immersing his head in water evoked extreme apprehension. His difficulties with the pool and with water became so troublesome that he found himself unable to even dangle his legs into water while sitting on the edge of the pool. This apprehension spread to the gym itself. The last time he went there, he had such an extreme panic reaction that the personnel at the gym called the police to remove him. The police arrived and Jordan refused to leave. A scuffle broke out and resulted in Jordan biting one of the officers. The police used a Taser on him, and he was taken to a jail cell. His sister was called to retrieve him. The police brought no charges as they saw Jordan as irrational and out of control.

Once in his sister's apartment, Jordan continued to be overwhelmed with panic and in an attempt to end his intense suffering, attempted to jump from a sixth story porch. His sister was able to convince him that he needed hospitalization. One the way to a well-known hospital in New York City, Jordan opened the car door, jumped out, and in what appeared to be a suicidal gesture, threw himself in front of oncoming cars. When questioned about this extreme act he claimed that he was not really trying to kill himself but rather trying to end the intense pain brought on by panic. It was clear to all that Jordan was progressively descending into irrational behavior and thought in reaction to the pain of his extended panic attacks.

It is difficult to accurately convey the intense level of suffering brought on by Jordan's panic. He has used the term, "seizure" to describe the sudden grip of intense fear that unpredictably but regularly fell upon him. During one of these "seizures" he would often thrash around maniacally, smashing objects and even hitting those who were nearby. At one point he punched his mother in the face and the next day, on seeing her blackened eye, asked if she had fallen. He had no memory of having hit her. It was clear that his panic attacks were rendering him an irrational, frightened, and crazed individual who was often unaware of what he was doing and who later had only minimal recall of what his behavior had wrought.

4. Secondary trauma

Before delving into Jordan's treatment, it is important to consider the impact that his extreme panic attacks had on his family. When an individual is traumatized as was Jordan, their emotional distress is transferred to those who have a close bond with that person. Typically, this group includes family members but can also include other caretakers such as therapists, physicians, nurses, etc. [4]. The process by which trauma is transferred from one individual to those who have a close and extended relationship with that person is referred to as secondary traumatization [5]. In Jordan's case his sister, who was a twin, and his mother who presumably spread Covid to her son, suffered the emotional pain of Jordan's distress. They felt powerless to alleviate his pain despite valiant efforts to coordinate treatment teams, find hopefully effective treatment facilities, and obtain a veritable army of occupational therapists, health aides, psychologists, psychiatrists, dieticians, and others. They clearly felt Jordan's pain and agonized over their inability to find some magical combination of therapeutic elements that would stop the suffering of their beloved family member. Jordan's sister would often take it upon herself to advise the physicians of the appropriate modes of treatment based upon her frenzied search of the internet. This proved to be counterproductive because after a while the physicians began to become defensive and non-responsive to her incessant questioning of their decisions. What she eventually came to understand was that Jordan's treatment team was not being negligent or uncaring but that they simply did not know how to alleviate Jordan's torturous panic attacks and his occasional thrashing both of which appeared to be brought on by the inflammation and oversensitivity of his ailing nervous system.

5. Psychological intervention

In general, panic attacks are treated both psychologically and pharmacologically [6] and this section will spotlight the former. Cognitive-behavioral therapy (CBT) interventions are often used, and these are frequently coupled with breathing techniques and meditation. Prior to engaging in interventions, it is important to assure the patient that panic disorder is a known phenomenon that afflicts approximately 2–5% of the general population [7], that a panic attack is not life threatening, and that it is often associated with feelings of extreme dread, trembling, extremity numbness, disorientation, hyperventilation, dizziness, and other symptoms. It is not uncommon for patients who experience panic attacks to fear that they might die or become insane. Assurance that these are common beliefs during a panic attack can be helpful in lessening the dread that the panic sufferer may encounter. It is also often helpful to provide the panic victim with information sources to reduce the chances of engaging in catastrophic thinking. This providing of information and perspective can be seen as cognitively oriented intervention that helps to allay extremely negative and fatalistic beliefs.

Another CBT intervention specifically targeted Jordan's tendency toward catastrophic thinking. In his case the catastrophizing involved the belief that "My life is over," "I will never get better." Jordan and I worked together in such a way that allowed him to understand that there was no evidence to support such a negativistic view, and that there was abundant evidence that people recover from AE based panic. Jordan was encouraged to engage in his own scientifically based skepticism of such thoughts and was generally able to do so. This technique was practiced between episodes of panic because once in the throes of a panic attack, logical and rational thinking are unavailable to most sufferers.

In Jordan's case a specific breathing exercise was also practiced that involved inhaling through the nose for 4 s, holding the breath for 5 s, and exhaling for 7 s. This exercise provided him with a tool to control the hyperventilation that he commonly experienced during a panic attack and reduced some the dizziness and tingling that were associated with this hyperventilation. He stated that the breathing exercise reduced the intensity of his panic but did not eliminate the disorder. He was clearly suffering but his pain was less than that which would normally be occurring without intervention. Unfortunately, it became apparent that unless I was guiding him in the controlled breathing exercise, he was unlikely to do it on his own. As I was unable to be with him daily to guide him through the breathing exercise, I taught the approach to his sister and mother with whom he spoke multiple times during the day. This helped considerably as they were able to get Jordan to engage in controlled breathing daily and often more than once during any given day.

Meditation techniques were coupled with the controlled breathing. Once Jordan had gained some level of control using the breathing techniques, a guided meditation was used. The meditation had to be guided because the concept of simply clearing his mind of intruding thoughts as is common in many forms of meditation, was beyond his capability given the ongoing panic disorder. One meditation that proved to be helpful was the "Mountain Meditation" [8] in that it provided the self-view of strength and imperviousness. The meditation is usually done in a sitting position where one directs one's attention to the characteristics of a mountain. One's lower extremities are viewed as the base of the mountain which is solid and imperturbable. The arms and shoulders are seen as projections from the mountain that are unchanged by winds, rain, or any other environmental events. The head as viewed as the top of the mountain that stands above and is unaffected by the travails and disturbances that people commonly encounter. The entire meditation takes approximately 20 min and emphasis is placed upon strength, endurance, and ability to be unmoved and unshaken. The images of strength and immobility help to counter the agitation and vulnerability commonly experienced by those enduring panic attacks. Other meditations were also used like the "Lake Meditation" which emphasizes stillness and tranquility [8]. Despite disturbances on the surface of the water, the lake ultimately returns to stillness and serenity. Imagining himself to have the characteristics of the lake helped Jordan to reduce his agitation.

A final form of psychological intervention for both Jordan and his family was supportive counseling. Jordan's illness seemed to come out of the blue and was terribly disruptive to him and extremely anxiety provoking to his mother and sister. Everyone seemed to benefit from encouragement and assurance that things would get better and that the brain had a natural tendency to move in the direction of self-repair and self-cure. A good example of this is the impressive recoveries made by those who have experienced brain damage due to strokes. Many of the functions lost to strokes are often recovered with various exercises that combine cognitive and physical activity. Jordan and his family were encouraged to read numerous anecdotal reports of people who recovered from the disability wrought by AE. These reports and the provision of emotional support went a long way in facilitating Jordan's eventual improvement.

6. Pharmacological, medical, and physiological intervention

When Jordan was first taken to the hospital following his initial irrational behaviors and attempts at self-injury, the hospital staff appeared to be at a loss. His doctors thought he had some form of psychosis and treated Jordan with antipsychotics, anti-anxiety and antidepression agents. The sedating effect that these medications resulted in some reduction of his anxious thrashing, but his panic disorder persisted, and he continued to verbalize the desire for his life to come to an end. The flailing about for some method of treating this agitated patient went on for several months until it was finally decided to do a spinal puncture. The results of this procedure led the involved neurologists and psychiatrists to conclude that he was suffering from autoimmune encephalitis. This diagnosis provided some direction for treatment, but the concept of a "cure" continued to be a distant hope.

Autoimmune encephalitis was first reported in the 1960s [9] and was initially described as limbic encephalitis (LE). LE encompassed symptoms including seizures, movement disorders, behavioral changes, mood disorders, cognitive impairment, and an altered level of consciousness. Except for the incoordination seen in movement disorders, Jordan appeared to be displaying all these symptoms. The disorder is now seen as affecting various brain structures, not just the limbic system, and is now termed AE or autoimmune encephalitis, a disorder involving the immune system's attack on various brain structures [10].

Having arrived at a diagnosis of AE, a twofold treatment was decided upon. The first was the use of steroids. The goal here was to reduce inflammation of the nervous system. The second line of attack was intravenous immunoglobulin (IVIG) infusion. The latter was aimed deactivating the immune system's attack on health neural tissue. Jordan received two such treatments of combined steroids and IVIG in the hope of a remission of his symptoms. However, the treatments not only proved ineffective in the short run, but it appeared that after the use of steroids his symptoms of agitation, panic, and thrashing became worse. Why this occurred is unclear because there were anecdotal reports from his treatment team that this intervention appeared to have reduced symptoms in other cases of AE that his physicians had encountered. On the other hand, there are researchers who report that available evidence shows that the combination of IVIG and steroid intervention continues to be ineffective for a significant number of patients suffering from AE [11]. The latter view certainly appeared to be valid in Jordan's case.

Given the obvious lack of progress in Jordan's behavior following two administrations of combined IVIG and steroids, the decision was made by his treatment team to

DOI: http://dx.doi.org/10.5772/intechopen.106138

provide him a second line of treatment called rituximab. Rituximab is a medication that is often used in the treatment of rheumatoid arthritis and is said to specifically inhibit B cells of the immune system. It is also used when the combined IVIG-steroid treatment fails stop the immune systems attack on healthy neural tissue that occurs in autoimmune encephalitis [12]. The rituximab treatment was done on two occasions approximately 6 weeks apart. One of the concerns voiced by Jordan's physicians was that because rituximab suppresses the immune system, the patient then becomes vulnerable to any potential infection to which he or she might be exposed. Jordan's treatment was taking place a time of increased infection rates of Covid in New York City so the concern for infection was realistic. In fact, the routine of the hospital was to isolate Jordan after the rituximab treatments. Visitors were required to be fully vaccinated, to wear masks, and to also wear latex gloves.

The idea that he might be immune compromised did nothing to help Jordan with his panic attacks. In the immediate aftermath of his rituximab treatments, he would be on the phone with his family all day. His sister once noted that that he had made approximately 150 calls on 1 day. Approximately 1 month after his last rituximab treatment, there did appear to be some diminishing of the intensity and frequency of Jordan's panic attacks. They were continuing to occur multiple time per day but there were periods, especially in the early afternoons, where he did seem to be less tormented by anxiety.

At around this time Jordan was transferred to another hospital in Yonkers, NY which specialized in the treatment of patients with specific neurological disorders such as encephalitis and traumatic brain injury. This hospital was one of the few placements that would accept him. The uncontrolled thrashing about and occasional breaking of objects in his hospital room during extreme panic attacks resulted in his being a patient that no one wanted in their facility. One novelty of his placement in Yonkers was that he was able to go outside unattended. He would occasionally go to a local basketball court to practice his shooting. Often the overstimulation of having been outside would precipitate a panic attack, so his increased freedom turned out to be a mixed blessing.

As a rule, physical exercise has beneficial effects on psychological and neurological functioning [13]. There is considerable speculation as to why this is the case but one of the more popular view sis known as the endorphin hypothesis [14]. Exercise is said to result in the release of the endogenous opiate beta-endorphin which is said to produce a calming effect on the nervous system and to result in mood elevation. The hypothesis is not without its critics who, among other critiques, note that beta endorphins do not cross the blood–brain barrier and therefore are unlikely to have an impact of neurological and psychological states. A competing hypothesis for the benefit of exercise is referred to as the endocannabinoid hypothesis [15]. Endocannabinoids, which are like the THC found in marijuana are released during exercise and are said to be capable of crossing the blood brain barrier. Regardless of theoretical view, it appears that in Jordan's case mild exercise such as shooting baskets or having a brief leisurely walk, proved beneficial in terms of reducing his level of panic, whereas more strenuous exercise had the opposite effect and precipitated intense panic reactions.

7. Transition to supportive care

Jordan was transferred to a private long-term care facility in Pennsylvania following his stay at the medical center in Yonkers, NY. At the time of his transfer Jordan had been in and out of various hospitals and neurological care facilities for 22 months. It was only at the time of his latest transfer that his panic attacks began to subside. He continued to be moderately anxious, depressed, and often felt overwhelmed, but the extreme panic disorder that he endured for almost 2 years, now appeared to be a torturous event of the past.

The question that arises is what was responsible for the reduction in his panic attacks. It is possible that the psychological supports and interventions that were put in place eventually took hold and helped Jordan deal with his anxieties. It is also possible that the medical interventions such as IVIG, steroids, and rituximab brought about the panic reductions by reducing the immune system's response and inflammation. Mild exercise and family support might also be pointed to as having been beneficial to him. However, if we objectively view what is known in Jordan's case, we must come to the somewhat unsettling conclusion that any of these interventions or some combination of them were what proved beneficial. It is also possible that none of them were responsible for change and that the brain's tendency to move in the direction of self-healing, as is seen in cases of stroke, is what eventually brought about change, e.g., [16]. This self-healing position suggests that, given sufficient time and effort to change one's behavior, the brain itself is the healing agent.

8. Conclusion

Jordan now resides in a supportive care facility where he has psychologists, psychiatrists, nurses, and recreational therapists. He is kept socially engaged and participates in both individual and group psychotherapy. He is receiving therapeutic doses of antianxiety and antidepression agents but no neuroleptics and no immune system targeted medications. His panic attacks have subsided and plans are to integrate him into the community by encouraging him to attend various social events and attempt to find employment. Given Jordan's background as a psychology professor, there is some discussion of having him provide counseling services to others within the supportive care facility. His training and difficult experiences with a severe case of neurologically induced panic, make him an ideal candidate for such a position.

Jordan views himself and his situation realistically. He sees himself as having endured the neurological torment of autoimmune encephalitis and that, for reasons unknown to him, he is beginning to recover. He is thankful that the panic that once gripped his life is no longer present. Each new day brings further improvements in terms of his willingness to engage in social events, to participate in therapeutic activities, and in his overall hopefulness that he will continue to improve to the point where he can get back to his former life. My impression, as one of his treating psychologists, is that he will not only be able to regain that which he once had, but that the traumatic experiences he has endured because of his illness will have given him greater depth and perspective. There is a possibility that his overall functioning may be better than it was prior to his illness. This is a relatively common outcome that is seen among those who have lived through various forms of trauma [17]. At this point, his treatment team is of the opinion that Jordan will make a complete recovery.

DOI: http://dx.doi.org/10.5772/intechopen.106138

Author details

Robert W. Motta
Hofstra University, Hempstead, NY, USA

*Address all correspondence to: motta9182@gmail.com

References

[1] American Psychiatric Association. Diagnostic and Statistical Manual of Mental Disorders. 5th ed. Washington, DC: American Psychiatric Association; 2013

[2] Younger D. The Autoimmune Brain. Rowman & Littlefield; 2019

[3] Butler D, Mosley GL. The Explain Pain Protectometer Handbook (8315). NOI Group; 2015

[4] McCann L, Pearlman LA. Vicarious traumatization: A framework for understanding the psychological effects of working with victims. Journal of Traumatic Stress. 1990;**3**:131-149

[5] Motta RW. Secondary trauma. International Journal of Emergency Mental Health. 2008;**10**:291-298

[6] Bystritsky A, Khalsa SS, Cameron ME, Schiffman J. Current diagnosis and treatment of anxiety disorders. Psychiatry Investigation. 2013;**38**:30-57

[7] Baxter AJ, Vos T, Scott KM, Ferrari AJ, Whitehead HA. The global burden of anxiety disorders. Psychological Medicine. 2010;**44**:2363-2374

[8] Kabat-Zinn J. Wherever You Go There You Are: Mindfulness Meditation in Everyday Life. New York: Hyperion; 1994

[9] Corsellis JA, Goldberg GJ, Norton AR. "Limbic encephalitis" and its association with carcinoma. Brain. 1968;**91**(3):481-496

[10] Saraya AW, Worachotsueptrakun K, Vutipongsatorn K, Sonpee C, Hemachudha T. Differences and diversity of autoimmune encephalitis in 77 cases of a single tertiary care center. BMC Neurology;**19**:273

[11] Yang J, Xueya L. Immunotherapy for refractory autoimmune encephalitis. Frontiers of Immunology. 2021;**12**:790962. DOI: 10.3389/fimmu.2021.790962

[12] Lancaster E. The diagnosis and treatment of autoimmune encephalitis. Journal of Clinical Neurology. 2016;**12**(1):1-13

[13] Manger TA, Motta RW. The impact of an exercise program on posttraumatic stress disorder, anxiety, and depression. International Journal of Emergency Mental Health. 2005;**7**:49-57

[14] Farrell PA, Gates WK, Mashud MG, Morgan WP. Increases in plasma beta-endorphin immunoreactivity after treadmill running in humans. Journal of Applied Physiology. 1982;**52**:1245-1249

[15] Smaga L, Bystrowska B, Gawlinski D, Przegalinski R, Filip M. The endocannabinoid/endovanilloid system and depression. Current Neuropharmacology. 2014;**12**:462-474

[16] van der Kolk BA. The Body Keeps the Score. New York, NY: Viking

[17] Tedeschi RG, Calhoun LG. Posttraumatic Growth: Conceptual Foundations and Empirical Evidence. Lawrence Earlbaum; 2004

Chapter 2

Perspective Chapter: Prevalence and Management of the Panic Disorder in Nepal

Bhupendra Singh Gurung

Abstract

Although panic attacks are not life-threatening, they can be terrifying and have a substantial impact on your quality of life. Treatment, on the other hand, can be quite effective. Little attention is paid to mental health in Nepal. There is no mental health law and the National Mental Health Policy formulated in 1997 has yet to come into full effect. Unspecified anxiety disorder (15.7%), adjustment disorder (13.9%), and post-traumatic stress disorder were the most frequently diagnosed conditions (8.3%). In 2018, the KCH CAP (OPD) cared for 2477 children, of whom 1529 were men and 948 were women. The most common diagnoses were anxiety disorder (524). Children ranging in age from 6 to 18 years old took part in the study. Nepal has one general hospital dedicated to mental illness and four private mental hospitals. Inpatient mental health care is provided primarily by 19 medical schools, 36 private-public hospitals, and many 27 public hospitals. The counseling situation in Nepal is largely poor. Advanced psychotherapy is provided by 35 clinical psychologists who are licensed practitioners in Nepal. In a 2018 research with 2477 individuals, 524 incidences of anxiety disorders were identified. Supervised counseling and psychotherapy practice is a relatively new concept in Nepal.

Keywords: anxiety disorder, panic disorder, prevalence, psychotherapy, and counseling

1. Introduction

In South Asia, between China and India, the Federal Democratic Republic of Nepal is a landlocked nation. Nepal has a varied topography, with the Tarai, or flat river plain, in the south, hilly areas in the center, and the high Himalayas in the north. The nation, which is divided into seven provinces (Pradesh), is a federal parliamentary republic, with Kathmandu serving as the capital [1].

In the general community, panic disorder is fairly prevalent. It is the anxiety illness that requires the most medical attention and is the most expensive in terms of mental health issues. The Diagnostic and Statistical Manual of Mental Health Disorders (DSM) describes a panic attack as "an abrupt rush of extreme dread or discomfort" that reaches a peak in a matter of minutes. A panic episode is accompanied by four or more of a certain set of physical symptoms. The frequency of panic episodes might range from several times per day to only a few times a year. Attacks happen suddenly, which is a defining characteristic of panic disorder. Often, there is no clear cause of the panic episode. Nepalese aged 16 to 40 suffer from mental health problems, with cases on the rise among children as Nepal conducts its first national mental health survey. Psychiatrists warn that various studies also show that mental health affects people of all ages [2]. Nepal's population has reached 29,192,480, with a 10.18% rise in the last 10 years [3].

A survey has found that 30% of Nepal's population suffers from psychiatric problems. Mental health is not well-recognized or taken seriously in Nepal. The government spends less than 1% of its total budget on healthcare in this area. Although precise data are not available on the prevalence of mental disorders in Nepal, small-scale studies have shown the prevalence to be as high as 37.5% in rural communities. In March 1995, the New Communist Party of Nepal (Maoist) ("CPN (Maoist)") began formulating a plan to launch an armed struggle, the so-called "People's War," against the government [3]. Nepal has seen a gradual increase in the incidence of depression, post-traumatic stress disorder, and suicide since the start of the conflict. Health experts estimate the rate of mental health problems in Nepal is as high as 30% [4].

On April 25, Nepal was hit by a magnitude 7.8 earthquake that caused severe damage to 1 of the country's 75 districts. Two weeks after that, on May 12, another magnitude 7.3 earthquake struck, worsening the humanitarian situation.

Common forms of stress shown in rapid assessments weeks after the Nepal earthquake included fear, anxiety, sadness, anger, sleep disturbances, and increased risk of suicide. Lockdowns, curfews, self-isolation, social distancing, and quarantines brought by the coronavirus disease and COVID-19 pandemic are impacting the overall physical, mental, and social health of Nepalese people. WHO Nepal Office (WCO) assisted the Minister of Health and Population (MoHP) in developing his COVID-19 Mental Health and Psychological Support (MHPSS) intervention framework. World Health Organization (WHO) helped develop the legal and policy framework for the implementation of the National Mental Health Strategy and Plan of Action developed by the Minister of Health and Population (MoHP). This includes required guidelines, standard operating procedures (SoPs), and training manuals [5].

1.1 Institutions

College courses and degrees in modern psychology began their journey to Nepal in the late 20th century at Tribhuvan University. Likewise, their professional training in modern clinical psychology in the form of a Master of Philosophy (M.Phil) in Clinical Psychology began in the late 1990s at the Institute of Medicine, Tribhuvan University (IOM/TU). It, therefore, felt essential to present the growth and development clearly and comprehensively in a clear and comprehensive manner. Specialization and continuing education in the form of fellowships, doctoral and postdoctoral programs, and competency-based training cover various forms of assessment, psychotherapy, neuropsychological approaches, integration with neuroscience, and specific therapeutic modalities, should focus on hyper-specialization in cross-cultural approaches, etc. Two years of M. Phil. in Clinical Psychology can be complemented by a Ph.D. in clinical psychology or the PsyD program. This is possible by setting up an independent clinical psychology department in each institute. More specialists are needed in areas, such as cognitive behavioral therapy, dialectical behavioral therapy, mindfulness-based therapies, couples and marriage therapies, family therapies, sexual therapies, drug and addiction therapies, rehabilitation, and supervision [6].

		#	Rate per 100,000
Generalist	Doctor	28,477[30]	96.0
	Nurse	27,040[31]	91.1
	Pharmacist	3761[32]	12.7
Specialist	Neurologist	25	0.1
	Psychiatrist	147	0.5
	Clinical psychologist	35	0.12
	Psychiatric Nurse	75	
	Lay counselors	~700	2.4

Table 1.
Human resource in mental health.

1.2 Human resources

There are about 147 psychiatrists and 3 child psychiatrists in Nepal. Of these, 110 work in the private sector. It is estimated that there are more than 75 psychiatric nurses and 30 private psychiatrists (**Table 1**). Almost all specialists are concentrated in large urban areas. There are also an estimated 700 nonprofessional consultants working in the public sector. Specialized training in psychiatry is offered at several institutions, while training in clinical psychology is offered at only one institution. As a result, about 15–20 psychiatrists are added each year, compared to only 2–3 clinical psychologists. However, Nepal does not have training programs for subspecialties, such as substance abuse, child mental health, or mental health for the elderly [7].

Despite the high exposure of CAP patients in daily practice, early career psychiatrists (ECPs) say they are not well trained and there is no standardized CAP course for ECPs in Nepal. The desire of the ECP to receive additional training from the CAP is very encouraging and positive [8]. Existing training in psychiatry may not be sufficient to provide meaningful psychotherapy training opportunities for most ECPs in Nepal. It is encouraging that most patients want to continue their psychotherapy training, and there is room for improvement in current psychotherapy training [9].

1.3 Healthcare facilities for mental health

Nepal has one general hospital dedicated to mental illness and four private mental hospitals. Inpatient mental health care is provided in 36 private hospitals and 27 public hospitals. There are also three outpatient services for children and adolescents. Nepal has adopted the mhGAP tools to fit its context, in the form of the Community Mental Health Care Package 2017. Anxiety is one of the common mental disorders included. A set of psychotropic medications, including antipsychotics, antidepressants, anxiolytics, mood stabilizers, and antiepileptics are available at health facilities of all levels across Nepal. Medicines are prescribed by registered medical doctors. However, health assistants employed in primary health care also prescribe after receiving training and following certain government protocols. Counseling on psychosocial is short-duration training. Usually, such training has a time duration of 6 months [10].

1.4 Psychosocial counseling and traditional practice

The historical point of counseling in Nepal has been recorded since the early 1990s. After Nepalese-speaking Bhutanese citizens were deported from Bhutan to Nepal between 1993 and 1996. Places of refuge required not only basic needs but also emotional support. This host country, Nepal, then began to see the importance of counseling after seeing many mental and psychosocial issues [8].

From priests and shamans to doctors with western training, the medical profession has always played a significant role in Nepal. These experts use a stethoscope or a ritual to evaluate the issue. Therapy claims to be able to quiet the mind through rituals or to treat illness with medications. Psychotherapists and counselors are viewed as devoted siblings who wish to hear their patients' ideas, sentiments, and feelings. To address the crises of torture survivors, the Center for Victims of Torture (CVICT) employs client-centered problem-solving counseling. In addition to focusing on human rights, CVICT also emphasizes client needs, goals, and ideals, as well as empowerment and self-reliance. Most individuals who are familiar with the idea of counseling think that it is all about providing consolation and guidance [11].

Little attention is paid to mental health in Nepal. There is no mental health law and the National Mental Health Policy formulated in 1997 has yet to come into full effect. The counseling situation in Nepal is largely poor. The training courses are usually short and do not involve clinical practice. Training is mostly given by foreign trainers who are new to the cultural environment. Counseling is commonly misunderstood, often resulting in judgmental and uninformed implementation and sometimes wrong practices. The state of counseling is further complicated by the arbitrary application of the word "counselor" to anyone doing social work within a non-governmental organization (NGO) setting. The five-month paraprofessional course begins with a 3-week core training phase, followed by multiple cycles of alternating supervised internships and continuing education courses for increasingly advanced skills and subjects. Working with western-oriented therapeutic assumptions in a non-Western setting requires adjustments to increase cultural relevance [12]. To create qualified counselors, the MA in counseling psychology was introduced in 2017 [13]. Cognitive behavioral therapy is mainly used to address psychological problems by clinical psychologists whereas client-centered counseling is practiced by counselors [14].

A group of gestalt therapists from Europe, formed a Gestalt Psychotherapy Institute in Kathmandu, Nepal. For a group of psychologists and counselors who work with children, refugees, and victims of sexual abuse and torture, the institute would offer psychotherapy and counseling in the area along with a Gestalt psychotherapy training program that adheres to the international standards of the EAGT (European Association for Gestalt Therapy) [15]. The Nepal Youth Foundation (NYF) launched a program called Sandplay Therapy. This has shown to be incredibly beneficial for the youngsters [16].

Supervised counseling and psychotherapy practice is a relatively new concepunderin Nepal. In Nepal, supervised counseling practice is still a novel idea. The majority of it is unsupervised. The study found that students nowadays are handicapped by the overwhelming volume of western study material and the excessively hierarchical supervision they get. The participants understood that the concept of contextualized supervision training had a surprising amount of power [17].

2. Prevalence and management

The planning of the National Mental Health Survey, Nepal started in November 2017 and was carried out in January 2019 and was carried out in all 7 provinces of Nepal from January 2019 to January 2020. The total sample size of the survey was 15,088, including 9200 adults (ages 18 and older) and 5888 youth (ages 13 to 17). The data collection tool consisted of a sociodemographic questionnaire, a translated and adapted Nepalese version of the MINI International Neuropsychiatric Interview (MINI) 7.0.2 for DSM-5, a questionnaire on pathways to obtaining care/help-seeking behavior, and a questionnaire on Barriers to Accessing Care Nursing Assessment (BACE). The overall response rate for adult participation was 96.8% [18].

Worldwide, 10–20% of children and adolescents suffer from mental problems, with 50% of all onsets happening by age 14 and 75% occurring by age 25. A sizeable portion of the population is at risk of developing a mental condition because 40% of Nepal's population is under the age of 18. Though previously largely disregarded by the health agenda, child and adolescent mental health concerns have lately come to attention in Nepal [19].

Before the pandemic, a number of studies were conducted on the prevalence of mental disorders in the Nepali population. A nationwide cross-sectional study conducted in 2013 among a representative sample of adults in Nepal using the Hospital Anxiety and Depression Scale (HADS) showed age and gender-adjusted point prevalence of anxiety of 16.2% [20].

A systematic review of studies on the mental health impact of the COVID-19 pandemic on the general population in different countries, including Nepal, showed relatively high rates of symptoms of anxiety, depression, post-traumatic stress disorder, mental distress, and stress [16]. Under this pretext, the psychosocial results of the Nepalese population should be examined. However, the effect of COVID-19 on psychosocial well-being in Nepal has now not been thoroughly studied (**Table 2**).

The outpatient clinic for Child and Adolescent Psychiatry (CAP) headed by Dr. Arun R. Kunwar has been operating at Kanti Children's Hospital (KCH) in Kathmandu since July 21, 2015. KCH is the first and only government children's hospital in Nepal to offer specialized services for children and CAP is one of the few specialized services operated in this hospital. In 2018, the KCH CAP (OPD) cared for 2477 children, of whom 1529 were men and 948 were women. The most common diagnoses were anxiety disorder (524). Children ranging in age from 6 to 18 years old took part in the study. Seventy eight of the patients were diagnosed with general anxiety disorder (GAD), and 65 with separation anxiety. Whereas 62 people were diagnosed with social anxiety, 52 with obsessive–compulsive disorder (OCD), 64 with panic disorder, and 60 with physical fear of damage [21].

2.1 Arm conflict and mental health in Nepal

In 2008, 720 people participated in this cross-sectional survey. In the sample, 27.5% of participants reached the criterion for depression, 22.9% for anxiety, and 9.6% for PTSD [22]. Shakya et al. 2011 indicated that many psychiatric disorders had a significant political stressor during armed conflict. The study was conducted with 50 participants. Almost all participants had somatic symptoms followed by anxiety symptoms [23].

Prevalence of mental disorders among adult participants aged 18 years and above

Disorders	Lifetime (95% CI)	Current (95% CI)
Any mental disorder	**10.0 (8.5–11.8)**	**4.3 (3.5–5.2)**
Mood disorders	**3.0 (2.5–3.7)**	**1.4 (1.1–1.8)**
Bipolar Affective Disorder	0.2 (0.1–0.5)	0.1 (0.1–0.3)
Major Depressive Disorder (MDD	2.9 (2.3–3.7)	1.0 (0.8–1.4)
Neurotic and Stress related disorders	**3.0 (2.5–3.6)**	
Panic Disorder	0.7 (0.6–0.9)	0.4 (0.3–0.5)
Generalized Anxiety Disorder	0.8 (0.6–1.1)	
Phobic Anxiety Disorder	0.2 (0.1–0.4)	
Obsessive Compulsive Disorder	0.2 (0.1–0.4)	
Post-Traumatic Stress Disorder	0.0 (0.0–0.2)	
Dissociative disorder	1.0 (0.7–1.4)	
Mental and behavioral problems due to psychoactive substance use		
Alcohol use disorder	4.2 (3.6–4.8)	
Other substance use disorder	0.2 (0.1–0.3)	
Schizophrenia, Schizotypal, and Delusional disorders	0.2 (0.1–0.3)	0.1 (0.1–0.3)
Antisocial personality disorder	0.1	
Somatic Symptom Disorder	0.5 (0.3–0.8)	

Table 2.
Prevalence of mental disorder among adult participants aged 18 years and above.

2.2 Major earthquake and mental health in Nepal

Little is known regarding what kind of psychological state disaster interventions are effective within the months following earthquakes in areas like the Asian nation. Given the inveterately disaster-prone context, communities should incline the mandatory tools to arrange for future natural hazards and to recover once disasters strike. With this in mind, a three-day integrated psychological state disaster response intervention for earthquake survivors in the Asian nation was designed. The community-based cluster intervention is culturally acceptable, includes header skills and community-building activities, and was tested employing a cluster comparison style. Social cohesion is related to psychological state symptoms, thus higher rates of depression and post traumatic stress disorder (PTSD) are related to lower social cohesion. Participation in a 3-day intervention ends up in a rise in disaster preparedness; a decrease in psychological state symptoms (depression, PTSD); and a rise in social cohesion. Six intervention teams, each with 20 participants, underwent the three-day psychological state integrated disaster readiness intervention at a similar time in every community. Six Nepali clinicians in the United Nations agency were experts in the native languages and were informed with the relevant subcultural team's junction rectifier **of** the groups—two in every case. All of them have between 2 and 6 years of expertise in community leadership. Their academic backgrounds ranged from a three-year degree in scientific discipline to a six-month message certificate. Senior members of the analysis team, like the

ICD 10 Code	ICD 10 Diagnosis	Male		Female		Total	
		N	%	N	%	N	%
F43.2	Adjustment Disorder	7	13.5	13	23.2	20	18.52
F41.9	Reaction to severe stress, unspecified	8	15.4	11	19.6	19	17.59
F10.3	Mental and Behavioral Disorder due to use of alcohol	10	19.2	2	3.6	12	11.11
F43.1	Post Traumatic Stress Disorder	4	7.7	5	8.9	9	8.33
F32.1	Depressive episode	6	11.5	3	5.4	9	8.33
F43.0	Acute Stress Reaction	4	7.7	4	7.1	8	7.41
F41.0	Panic Disorder	4	7.7	3	5.4	7	6.48
F20	Schizophrenia	3	5.8	2	3.6	5	4.63
F23.0	Acute and Transient Psychotic Disorder	2	3.8	3	5.4	5	4.63
F41.1	Generalized Anxiety Disorder	1	1.9	4	7.1	5	4.63
F45.1	Undifferentiated Somatoform Disorder	2	3.8	1	1.8	3	2.78
F44.5	Dissociative (conversion) Disorder	0	0.0	2	3.6	2	1.85
G44.2	Tension-Type Headache	0	0.0	2	3.6	2	1.85
F33	Recurrent Depressive Disorder	1	1.9	0	0.0	1	0.93
G43	Migraine Headache	0	0.0	1	1.8	1	0.93
	Total	56	100	52	100	108	100

Table 3.
Disorder diagnosed during the visit to hospital.

second author, a doctorial level social worker/psychologist, and United Nations agency additionally provided on-the-spot oversight throughout implementation and educated facilitators over the fortnight. The temporary group-based intervention is also scaled up to be used not solely in the Asian nation but also in different nations that usually expertise earthquakes and different natural disasters [24].

Unspecified anxiety disorder (15.7%), adjustment disorder (13.9%), and post-traumatic stress disorder were the most frequently diagnosed conditions (8.3%) shown in **Table 3** [19]. Ten papers were identified, all involving 7876 participants. Two studies reported post-traumatic stress symptoms 10.7–**51%** prevalence of 10.7–**51%** in earthquake-affected children and adolescents in the Kathmandu district of Nepal. Another study reported that 53.2% of former child soldiers achieved the cut-o score for PTSD. The clinical prevalence of anxiety disorders has been reported as 18.8 to 24.4%, in different clinical samples of children and adolescents [25].

2.3 COVID-19 pandemic and mental health in Nepal

Utilizing a multistage proportionate stratified random selection method, a cross-section web-based study design was conducted with 422 Nepalese individuals in the provinces of Bagmati, Gandaki, and Lumbini (**Table 4**). To measure the severity of

SN	Province	District	Total Population from 18 and above according to census 2011	Sample
1	**Province number 3 (Bagmati)**	Kathmandu,	1,329,799	143
2	**Province 3**	Lalitpur	356,023	38
3	**Province 3**	Chitwan	408,976	44
4	**Gandaki Province**	Baglunj	171, 841	19
5	**Gandaki Province**	Syangja	194,696	21
6	**Gandaki Province**	Kaski	349,893	38
7	**Province 5**	Rupandehi	580,688	63
8	**Province 5**	Palpa	171,212	18
9	**Province 5**	Dang	353,171	38
		Total	3,916,299	422

Table 4.
Sample size of each district.

depression, stress, and anxiety, the DASS-21 tool was employed. Only 77.5% of whom reported experiencing no stress during lockdown experienced extremely high levels of anxiety [26].

There has been a negative impact on children and adolescents' (C&A) access to mental health care throughout Nepal. The mental health of C&A has been impacted by factors, such as school closures, home confinement, lockdowns, transportation issues, uncertainty, disruption of routine, and fear of infection. A suitable strategy to meet these objectives is an online platform. With this in mind, a multi-tiered children and adolescent mental health (CAMH) intervention model was created. It makes use of an online platform to train mental health professionals throughout Nepal, who would then organize sessions for C&A, teachers, parents, and caregivers and connect them to local and remote CAMH services via tele-consultation. With the goal of reaching 40,000 C&A, parents, teachers, and caregivers, this began as a trial program in June 2020 and will run through the end of February 2021. By November 2020, 1415 sessions had been successfully completed using this technique.

Reaching 28,597 people, out of them, 12,026 are parents, teachers, and caregivers from all 7 provinces of Nepal, making up 16,571 child and adolescent (C&A). The multi-tier intervention has been described in this research as a workable approach for resource-constrained settings and low middle-income countries (LMIC) like Nepal. It addresses the COVID-19-related CAMH problems [27].

2.4 Management

Similar to Western ethnopsychology, Nepali ethnopsychology (**Figure 1**) offers various divisions of the self (see **Figure 1**). The physical body (Nepali: jiu or saarir), heart-mind (man), brain-mind (dimaag), spirit (saato), soul (atma), and one's social standing (ijjat) are the primary components. The family (pariwaar), which includes the extended family, and the spiritual realm, particularly connections with one's ancestors' deities, are additional significant divisions (kuldevta) (**Table 5**). The heart-mind and the brain-mind are important subjects in the treatment of mental illness. Memory and emotion are stored in the heart-mind. Psychotherapies including

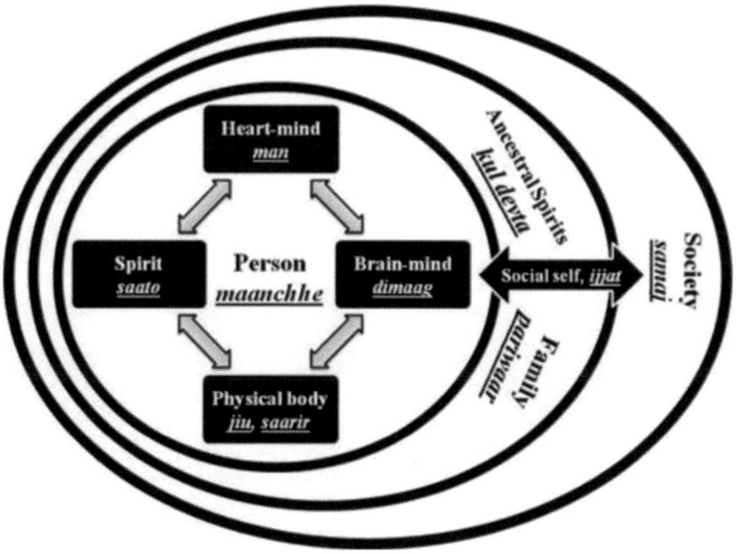

Figure 1.
Nepali ethnopsychological model of the self.

Ethno-psychology Component	Description	Cognitive Behavior Therapy (CBT)	Interpersonal Therapy (IPT)	Dialectical Behavior Therapy (DBT)
Heat-mind (*man*)	Organ of emotions, memories, and desire	'Feelings' in CBT should reference heart-mind processes	Heart-mind processes are examined in the context of social relationships; IPT grief theme relates to the heart-mind	Radical acceptance and change framed in heart-mind and brain-mind conflicts
Brain-mind (*dimaag*)	Organ of social responsibility and behavioral control	"Thoughts" and "appraisals" in CBT should reference brain-mind processes	Behavioral control through the brain-mind is examined in the context of social relationships	Brain-mind and heart-mind conflicts are reduced; the brain-mind is responsible for regulating "opposite actions" and "response prevention"
Physical body (*jiu, saarir*)	Physical sense organ, topography of pain	Somatic complaints in CBT may be consequence of heart-mind and brain-mind processes	The connection between physical suffering and relationships is explored through the social world, heart-mind, and physical body	"Opposite actions" and "response prevention" are used to prevent self-injury to the body

Ethno-psychology Component	Description	Cognitive Behavior Therapy (CBT)	Interpersonal Therapy (IPT)	Dialectical Behavior Therapy (DBT)
Spirit (*saato*)	Vitality, energy, and immunity to illness	Lost vitality in CBT can be associated with strong emotions in heart-mind (anger, fear)	Loss of vitality can be tied to difficulties in interpersonal relationships with both family and ancestral spirits	Preventing soul loss (*saato jaane*) is addressed by reducing intensity of emotions in heart-mind
Social status (*ijjat*)	Personal and family social standing and respect	Social status can be maintained through better insight into thoughts and feelings in CBT	Social status is explored by considering network of relationships; interpersonal deficits related to perceived social status can be challenged	Distress from perceived social status loss (*bejjat*) is managed through heart-mind emotional acceptance
Family and community relationships	Social support and social burden	The brain-mind processes related to relationships are explored for their effect on heart-mind processes	IPT themes of interpersonal disputes and role transitions examine social relationships	The group therapy component of DBT is used to discuss and model appropriate social relationships

Table 5.
Components of Nepali ethnopsychology in therapy modalities.

cognitive behavior therapy, interpersonal therapy, and dialectical behavior therapy can all benefit from the use of Nepali ethnopsychology. Any of these ways must have an excellent therapist who simultaneously doubles as an ethnographer [28].

The CVICT personnel received training in the Emotional Freedom Technique (EFT), a novel form of therapy, in 1997. This therapy is based on the idea that disturbances in the energy field are what trigger unfavorable feelings. It is a streamlined variation of Thought Field Therapy (TFT) that was created by Gary Craig. It is quite easy to use. Focusing on the issue while lightly touching an acupuncture meridian constitutes this technique. A year later, eye movement desensitization and reprocessing (EMDR) was introduced. A therapy for PTSD that has been empirically demonstrated to be successful (these are post-trauma symptoms, which include nightmares, palpitation, fear, intrusive thoughts, anger, re-experiencing, and bodily pains). These techniques were successfully used for excessive fears, traumatic memories, anxiety, depression, medically unexplained pain, and guilt. There have been cases where one resolved issue leads to another chain of issues, which are treated during consecutive visits [29].

To provide therapeutic recovery to the Bhutanese refugees in Nepal, a community-based group intervention was started. During the Maoist insurgency, group therapy was further utilized and expanded to include war victims in the post-conflict period. Out of several interventions, the International Committee of the Red Cross (ICRC)'s Hateymalo Program, the Problem Management Plus (PM+) group therapy model from the World Health Organization (WHO), Group Interpersonal Therapy (IPT) for teenagers, Dialectical Behavioral Therapy in Nepali (DBT-N) in minority women groups, and Common Thread (sajha-dhago) for women were some of the programs examined [30].

In order to prioritize mental, neurological, and drug use problems, the World Health Organization (WHO) introduced the mental health Gap Action Program (mhGAP) in 2008. The goal of mhGAP is to make it easier for nonspecialized healthcare professionals to deliver evidence-based interventions in basic healthcare settings. In addition, mhGAP promotes expanding access to mental health services by integrating mental health into primary healthcare [31].

2.5 Management in earthquake

In a resource-constrained rural Nepali setting, this research discusses the manualized, cross-cultural adaption of traditional dialectical behavior therapy (DBT) employing an iterative, collaborative, and phasic process approach. It was conducted with one particular subcultural group in rural Nepal, which was identified by its location, its religious preferences, its gender, and its line of work [32].

Tribhuvan University Teaching Hospital [13] promptly developed a 24-hour critical incident crisis management help center, and bed-to-bed psychological assistance was offered in the triage rooms and wards. PFA, trauma therapy, and appropriate psychiatric and nursing care were all delivered immediately by psychiatrists, clinical psychologists, nurses, and residents. The majority of the clients had anxiety disorders, including acute stress reaction (ASR) (44%), acute stress disorder (ASD) (9%), and anxiety disorders not otherwise specified (NOS) (18%). There was counseling for trauma, trauma-focused CBT, and behavioral treatments [33].

2.6 Trauma-focused therapies

A team of local nonspecialist mental health volunteers was trained to identify survivors with PTSD using the PTSD checklist for the Diagnostic and Statistical Manual of Mental Disorders, Fifth Edition. They were trained to deliver either shortened versions of narrative exposure therapy (NET)-revised or group-based control-focused behavioral treatment (CFBT). All adult survivors (aged 18 and above) in Bhaktpur fulfilling the DSM-5 criteria for PTSD were randomly offered either individual NET-R or group CFBT over a period of 2 weeks at the survey base hotel.

Therapists were offered daily on-site supervision by the trainers. All 58 participants who had received a provisional diagnosis of PTSD were randomly split into two groups, with 29 receiving individual NET-R treatments and the other half receiving group CFBT twice, 2 weeks apart. According to the results of the study, CFBT groups based on self-help manuals may be more suitable for rural populations with lower levels of education. Local mental health personnel can be taught brief trauma therapy quickly [34].

2.7 Psychosocial management in COVID-19

With cooperation with the Nepal Association of Clinical Psychologists, WCO also assisted in the national adaptation and translation of the International Federation of the Red Cross Guideline on Remote Psychological First Aid. This publication acted as a manual for adapting the psychosocial support delivery to the particular issues faced by the epidemic. This procedure for delivering PFA remotely was explained to at least 120 counselors [34]. Since the COVID-19 pandemic, it is anticipated that mental problems including depression and anxiety would become more common. Together with the Nepal Association of Clinical Psychologists, the WHO/International Committee of the Red Cross Guideline of Psychological First Aid was also translated and modified for the local environment. More than 40,000 people received psychosocial support in some way; more than 20,000 children and adolescents were offered crucial mental health support; and WHO Country Office for Nepal also hosted regular meetings (mental health subcluster meetings) to coordinate activities among partners. As a result of coordinated efforts, these outcomes were achieved [35].

2.8 The multi-tiered CAMH intervention model

In this intervention model, COVID-19 has been taken as one of the stressors that could adversely affect CAMH. The model incorporates basic psychosocial support for management of stress, tailored more toward COVID-19 related stress, but is not limited to it. This also includes identification and management of CAMH problems locally, and remotely through link with tele-consultation services. The same framework can be used for management of CAMH issues due to other stressors as well. This is a multi-tier model because it includes training of mental health professionals by master trainers through Training of Trainers (TOTs) sessions intervention model, COVID-19 has been taken as one of the stressors that could adversely affect CAMH. The model incorporates basic psychosocial support for management of stress, tailored more toward COVID- 19 related stress, but is not limited to it. This also includes identification and management of CAMH problems locally, and remotely through a link with tele-consultation services. The same framework can be used for management of CAMH issues due to other stressors as well. This is a multi-tier model because it includes training of mental health professionals by master trainers through Training of Trainers (TOTs) sessions (**Figure 2**). The strategy includes fundamental psychological assistance for stress management, albeit it is not just for COVID-19-related stress. This also involves local and distant

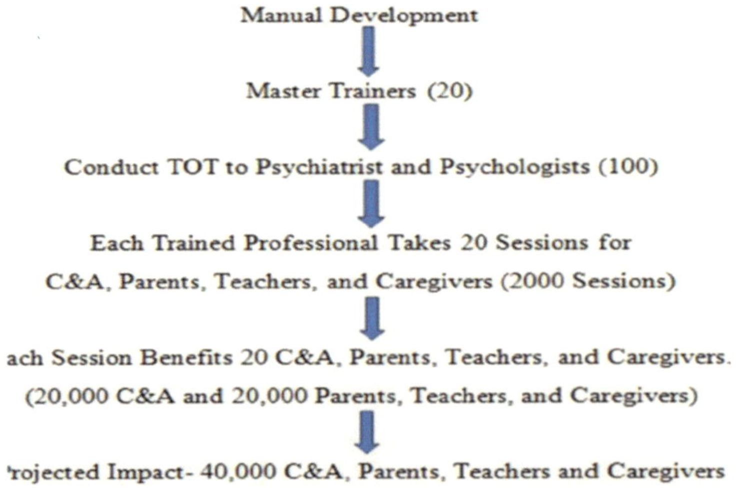

Figure 2.
Flowchart of multi-tiered CAMH intervention phases.

management of CAMH issues via connections to teleconsultation services. The same strategy was applied to managing CAMH symptoms brought on by additional stresses. This strategy has several levels (**Table 6**) since it includes the training of mental health professionals by master trainers through Training of Trainers (TOT) sessions, and the TOT recipients will then lead sessions with C&A, parents, teachers, and other caregivers.

The incorporation of psychotherapy in psychiatric training was noted by more than two-thirds of ECPs. The majority (67.6%) stated that it required training, while the majority (45%) stated that it only covers theoretical topics. About one-third had expertise in psychotherapy training, mostly in cognitive-behavioral treatment (CBT) (**Table 7**) [36].

It was considerably less frequent to have experience with interpersonal, family, or other treatments. **Table 8**, shows that among those who had received psychotherapy training, just half were happy with it. The duration of their psychiatric monitoring, which was stated to be elective by 50% of those who received it, was reportedly less than 50 hours [36].

Tiers	Description
One	Children and adolescents in different parts of Nepal
Two	Parents, Teachers, and Caregivers in different parts of Nepal.
Three	Mental health professionals: psychiatrists and psychologists working in different parts of Nepal. They have an MD degree in Psychiatry or Master's degree in Psychology. Their work includes mental health services primarily targeting adults.
Four	Child and Adolescent Psychiatry team at Kanti Children's Hospital. This comprises a team of child and adolescent psychiatrists, and clinical psychologists. They have post-MD degrees of specialization in Child and Adolescent Psychiatry and Post-master's degrees of specialization in clinical psychology, respectively. This team exclusively works in the field of CAMH.

Table 6.
Multi-tiered CAMH intervention.

Demographic details and psychotherapy training status of respondents (*n* = 51)	
Demographic details	
Gender	Male: 58.8% (*n* = 30)
Age	Mean 31.3 years (± 3.4)
Job position	Psychiatry trainee: 37.3% (*n* = 19)
	General adult psychiatrist: 58.8% (*n* = 30)
	Child psychiatrist: 3.9% (*n* = 2)
Psychotherapy training in Nepal	
Is psychotherapy included in your psychiatry training?	Yes: 72.5% (*n* = 37)
Mandatory (*v*. Optional)	Mandatory: 67.6% (*n* = 25)
Theoretical (*v*. Practical)	Theoretical: 78.4% (*n* = 29)

Table 7.
Demographic details and psychotherapy training.

Respondents' experiences in psychotherapy training (n = 51)	
Have you done any training in psychotherapy?	
No, have not trained in psychotherapy	64.7% (n = 33)
Yes, currently training	29.4% (n = 15)
Yes, completed training	5.9% (n = 3)
If Yes, which modality? (n = 18)	Cognitive-behavioral therapy: 94.4% (n = 17)
	Interpersonal therapy: 50% (n = 9)
	Family therapy: 38.9% (n = 7)
	Psychodynamic therapy: 22.2% (n = 4)
	Group therapy: 5.6% (n = 1)
	Motivational enhancement therapy: 5.6% (n = 1)
Have you undergone personal psychotherapy?	Yes: 3.9% (n = 2)
Psychotherapy supervision	
Access to supervision	66.6% (n = 12)
Mandatory (*v*. Optional)	Optional: 58.3% (n = 7)
Format of supervision (n = 12)	Individual: 41.6% (n = 5)
	Group: 25% (n = 3)
	Mixed: 33.3% (n = 4)
Duration of supervision (n = 12)	<50 h: 58.3% (n = 7)
	50–100 h: 16.7% (n = 2)
	>100 h: 25% (n = 3)
Satisfaction with psychotherapy training (n = 18)	
	Dissatisfied: 22.2% (n = 4)
	Satisfied: 50% (n = 9)
	Neither satisfied nor dissatisfied: 27.8% (n = 5)

Table 8.
Respondent's experience in psychotherapy.

3. Conclusions

Since the war, a significant earthquake, and the COVID-19 epidemic, there have been increased reports of mental health problems. Panic disorder is one of the most prevalent mental health conditions. In addition to DSM-5, ICD-10 is the diagnostic code most frequently employed by practitioners. Panic disorder is one of the conditions that is frequently identified. Patients with panic disorder get both medication treatment and psychotherapy, as well as deep breathing exercises and progressive muscular relaxation. Cognitive behavior therapy is the therapy that is used the most frequently. A research report generally does not contain case studies of recognized panic disorder. Although there is a specific study on other problems, such as substance use disorders, schizophrenia, mood disorders, anxiety, and depression. On the subject of panic disorder particularly, the little study is done. In the country's capital, there is a greater concentration of mental health services. Access to the service might be challenging for people who live in rural locations. As a result, there is a great probability that they will not receive proper care in addition to the traditional healer. Small-scale surveys and one nationwide survey both demonstrate the prevalence of panic disorder. However, there is relatively little research done on counseling and psychotherapy. The need for psychotherapeutic management is growing at the moment, but there is a lack of public awareness. Long-term treatment built on academic training should be implemented as part of national health policy. More resources and attention should be devoted to mental health in Nepal than are currently being done.

Acknowledgements

The author would like to thank Dr. Arun Raj Kunwar MD, Head of Child and Adolescent Psychiatry Mental Health (CAPMH) Unit, Kanti Children's Hospital, Dr. Jasmin Ma MD, Project Manager, Child and Adolescent Psychiatry Mental Health (CAPMH) Unit, Kanti Children's Hospital, Child Workers in Nepal Concerned Centre (CWIN), Dr. Binod Dangal MD, Pasupati Chaulagain Memorial Hospital, and the team of Nepalese Association of Clinical Psychology.

Conflict of interest

"The authors declare no conflict of interest."

Appendices and nomenclature

#	Number
ASD	Acute Stress Disorder
ASR	Acute Stress Reaction
BACE	Barriers to Accessing Care Nursing Assessment
CPN	Communist Party of Nepal
COVID-19	Corona Virus Disease-2019
CAP	Child and Adolescent Psychiatry
C&A	Child and Adolescent
CFBT	Control-Focused Behavioral Treatment
CVICT	Centre for Victims of Torture
CWIN	Child Workers in Nepal Concerned Centre
DBT	Dialectical Behavior Therapy
DBT-N	Dialectical Behavioral Therapy in Nepali
DSM-5	Diagnostic and Statistical Manual of Mental Health Disorders-5
EAGT	European Association for Gestalt Therapy
ECPs	Early Career Psychiatrists
EFT	Emotional Freedom Technique
EMDR	Eye Movement Desensitization and Reprocessing
GAD	General Anxiety Disorder
HADS	(Hospital Anxiety and Depression Scale
ICD	International Classification of Diseases
ICRC	International Committee of the Red Cross
IOM/TU	Institute of Medicine, Tribhuvan University
IPT	Interpersonal Therapy

KCH	Kanti Children's Hospital
LMIC	Low Middle Income Countries
MA	Master of Arts
MoHP	Minister of Health and Population
MINI	International Neuropsychiatric Interview
M. Phil.	Master of Philosophy
mhGAP	Mental Health Gap Action Programme
NET	Narrative Exposure Therapy
NYF	Nepal Youth Foundation
NGO	Non-Governmental Organization
NOS	Not otherwise specified
OCD	Obsessive Compulsive Disorder
OPD	Outpatient Department
PM+	Problem Management Plus
PhD	Doctor of Philosophy
PsyD	Doctor of Psychology degree
MHPSS	Mental Health and Psychological Support
PTSD	Post Traumatic Stress Disorder
PTSD checklist	Post Traumatic Stress Disorder Checklist
SoPs	Standard Operating Procedures
TFT	Thought Field Therapy
TOTs	Training of Trainers
WCO	WHO Nepal Office
WHO	World Health Organization

Author details

Bhupendra Singh Gurung
Children and Adolescents Psychiatry Mental Health (CAPMH) Unit, Kanti Children's Hospital, Pasupati Chaulagain Memorial Hospital, Kathmandu, Nepal

*Address all correspondence to: tamubhupendra@gmail.com

References

[1] Available from: https://www.herd.org.np/uploads/frontend/Publications/PublicaPtionsAttachments1/1480578193-Mental%20Health%20in%20Nepal%20-%20A%20Backgrounder.pdf [7/19/2022]

[2] Available from: https://kathmandupost.com/valley/2018/10/10/22m-nepalis-suffer-from-mental-health-disorder [7/19/2022]

[3] Available from: https://kathmandupost.com/national/2022/01/27/nepal-s-population-is-29-192-480 [7/31/2022]

[4] Available from: https://www.ohchr.org/sites/default/files/Documents/Countries/NP/OHCHR_ExecSumm_Nepal_Conflict_report2012.pdf [7/25/2022]

[5] Available from: https://reliefweb.int/report/nepal/nepal-earthquake-humanitarian-response-april-september-2015 [7/26/2022]

[6] Available from: https://www.who.int/about/accountability/results/who-results-report-2020-mtr/country-story/2020/nepal-mental-health#:~:text=More%20than%204%25%20of%20Nepal's,worsened%20after%20COVID%2019%20pandemic. [7/31/2022]

[7] Rana M, Shakya S, Towards professional training in clinical psychology in Nepal. 2022. Available from: https://www.researchgate.net/publication/360216615_Towards_professional_training_in_clinical_psychology_in_Nepal. [7/29/2022]

[8] Available from: https://cdn.who.int/media/docs/default-source/mental-health/special-initiative/who-special-initiative-country-report---nepal---2022.pdf?sfvrsn=714028db_3&download=true [7/31/2022]

[9] Karki U, Rai Y, Dhonju G, Sharma E, Jacob P, Kommu J, et al. Child and adolescent psychiatry training in Nepal: Early career psychiatrists' perspective. Child and Adolescent Psychiatry and Mental Health. 2020. pp. 3-5. DOI: 10.1186/s13034-020-00319-5

[10] Rai, Y, Karki U, Mariana Pinto da C. Psychotherapy training in Nepal: Views of early career psychiatrists. BJPsych International. 2020;18:1-4. DOI: 10.1192/bji.2020.50. Available from: https://www.researchgate.net/publication/347065466_Psychotherapy_training_in_Nepal_views_of_early_career_psychiatrists [7/29/2022]

[11] Poudyal B. Using psychotherapy with torture survivors in Nepal. This article is a narrative about challenges in providing psychotherapy to victims of torture in Nepal, and how "power therapies" like EMDR, and EFT were helpful. 1999. Available from: https://www.researchgate.net/publication/342436204_Using_Psychotherapy_with_Torture_Survivors_in_Nepal

[12] Available from: https://www.researchgate.net/publication/225558486_Psychosocial_Counselling_in_Nepal_Perspectives_of_Counsellors_and_Beneficiaries#pfb [7/27/2022]

[13] Available from: https://www.rojimaharjan.com/2019/06/counseling-history-in-nepal.html [7/31/2022]

[14] Available from: https://sujenman.wordpress.com/2010/04/25/clinical-psychology-mental-health-in-nepal/ [8/1/2022]

[15] Available from: https://www.britishgestaltjournal.com/features/2018/3/19/frans-meulmeester-on-gestalt-therapy-in-nepal [8/1/2022]

[16] Available from: https://www.taylorfrancis.com/chapters/edit/10.4324/9781315656748-4/sandplay-therapy-nepal-chhori-laxmi-maharjan [8/1/2022]

[17] Saunders JM. Building bridges: Contextualising a counscounselinrvision course in Nepal and its potential impact on international practice. Counselling and Psychotherapy Research. 2022;**22**: 1-11. DOI: 10.1002/capr.12459

[18] Available from: http://nhrc.gov.np/publication/national-mental-health-survey-nepal-2020-factsheets-adults/ [7/28/2022]

[19] Chaulagain A, Kunwar A, Watts S, Guerrero A, Skokauskas N. Child and adolescent mental health problems in Nepal: A scoping review. International Journal of Mental Health Systems. 2019. p. 13. DOI: 10.1186/s13033-019-0310-y. Available from: https://www.researchgate.net/publication/335127340_Child_and_adolescent_mental_health_problems_in_Nepal_A_scoping_review

[20] Gautam K, Adhikari RP, Gupta AS, et al. Self-reported psychological distress during the COVID-19 outbreak in Nepal: Findings from an online survey. BMC Psychology. 2020;**8**:127. DOI: 10.1186/s40359-020-00497-z

[21] Luitel N, Jordans M, Sapkota R, Tol W, Kohrt B, Thapa S, et al. Conflict and mental health: A cross-sectional epidemiological study in Nepal. Social Psychiatry and Psychiatric Epidemiology. 2012. p. 48. DOI: 10.1007/s00127-012-0539-0. Available from: https://www.researchgate.net/publication/229013196_Conflict_and_mental_health_A_cross-sectional_epidemiological_study_in_Nepal

[22] Available from: DOI: 10.3126/hren.v9i2.4975 [7/31/2022]

[23] Welton-Mitchell C, James LE, Khanal SN, et al. An integrated approach to mental health and disaster preparedness: A cluster comparison with earthquake earthquake-affecteds in Nepal. BMC Psychiatry. 2018;**18**:296. DOI: 10.1186/s12888-018-1863-z 7/26/2022

[24] Shakya S, Psychiatric morbidity pattern in a patient after earthquake an at Tribhuvan University Teaching Hospital Nepal. Journal of the Institute of Medicine. 2017. p. 39. Available from: https://www.researchgate.net/publication/324223472_Psychiatric_morbidity_pattern_in_patient_after_earthquake_at_Tribhuvan_University_Teaching_Hospital_Nepal [7/29/2022]

[25] Basnet S, Bhandari B, Gaire B, Sharma P, Shrestha RM. Depression, stress and anxiety among residents of Nepal during COVID-19 Lockdown. Journal of Advanced Academic Research. 2021;**8**(1):53-62

[26] Karki U, Dhonju G, Rai Y, Kunwar A. Child and Adolescent Mental Health in Nepal. 2019. p. 30. Available from: https://www.researchgate.net/publication/335789345_Child_and_Adolescent_Mental_Health_in_Nepal. [7/28/2022]

[27] Kohrt B, Maharjan S, Timsina D, Griffith J. Applying Nepali ethnopsychology to psychotherapy for the treatment of mental illness and prevention of suicide among Bhutanese refugees. Annals of Anthropological Practice. 2012. p. 36. DOI: 10.1111/j.2153-9588.2012.01094.x. Available from:

https://www.researchgate.net/publication/264726087_Applying_Nepali:ethnopsychology_to_psychotherapy_for_the_treatment_of_mental_illness_and_prevention_of_suicide_among_Bhutanese_refugees [8/1/2022]

[28] Available from: https://www.researchgate.net/publication/342436204_Using_Psychotherapy_with_Torture_Survivors_in_Nepal

[29] Adhikari Y, Group Therapeutic Interventions in Nepal: Review of Research and Practices. 2022. Available from: https://www.researchgate.net/publication/360141999_Group_Therapeutic_Interventions_In_Nepal_Review_Of_Research_And_Practices

[30] mhGAP Intervention Guide for Mental, Neurological and Substance Use Disorders in Non-Specialized Health Settings: Mental Health Gap Action Programme (mhGAP). Geneva: World Health Organization; 2010. Available from: https://www.ncbi.nlm.nih.gov/books/NBK138690/

[31] Ramaiya MK, Fiorillo D, Regmi U, Robins CJ, Kohrt BA. A cultural adaptation of dialectical behavior therapy in Nepal. Cognitive and Behavioral Practice. 2017;24(4):428-444. DOI: 10.1016/j.cbpra.2016.12.005. PMID: 29056846; PMCID: PMC5645023. [7/27/2022]

[32] Rana M. Issues and challenges of Nepal earthquake 2015 on mental health services. 2016. Available from: https://www.researchgate.net/publication/336936782_Issues_and_Challenges_of_Nepal_Earthquake_2015_on_Mental_Health_Services

[33] Jha A et al. Identification and treatment of Nepal 2015 earthquake survivors with posttraumatic stress disorder by nonspecialist volunteers: An exploratory cross-sectional study. Indian Journal of Psychiatry. 2017;**59**(3):320-327. DOI: 10.4103/psychiatry.IndianJPsychiatry_236_16 7/26/2022

[34] Available from: https://www.who.int/about/accountability/results/who-results-report-2020-mtr/country-story/2020/nepal-mental-health#:~:text=More%20than%204%25%20of%20Nepal's,worsened%20after%20COVID%2019%20pandemic

[35] Available from: https://www.who.int/nepal/news/detail/07-04-2021-addressing-the-mental-health-needs-of-the-nepali-people-during-the-covid-19-pandemic [7/26/2022]

[36] Dhonju G, Kunwar A, Karki U, Devkota N, Bista I, Sah R. Identification and management of covid-19 related child and adolescent mental health problems: A multi-tier intervention model. Frontiers in Public Health. 2021. p. 8. DOI: 10.3389/fpubh.2020.590002. Available from: https://www.researchgate.net/publication/349047801_Identification_and_Management_of_COVID-19_Related_Child_and_Adolescent_Mental_Health_Problems_A_Multi-Tier_Intervention_Model

Section 2

Panic in Childhood and Work Settings

Chapter 3

Pediatric Panic Disorder, Review of Art Therapy as Supportive and Palliative Intervention

Kaveh Moghaddam

Abstract

A panic attack is defined as an episode of intense fear and anxiety including both physical symptoms and fearful thoughts. Panic disorder (PD) is diagnosed when a child has recurring panic attacks and ongoing concern about having more attacks for longer than 1 month. Children and teens with panic disorder sometimes avoid going places or avoid engaging in activities out of fear that a panic attack might occur. Although individual panic attacks are common, panic attacks that occur repeatedly are rare. They typically happen in only one to three percent of children and teens. Panic disorder usually does not affect children before the teenage years. Palliative and supportive interventions such as art therapy and family-based interventions are approaches that can help to reduction of this disorder's symptoms, especially in children and teens. In this chapter, these issues will be illustrated and the practical methods will be presented.

Keywords: panic disorder, palliative and supportive interventions, art therapy, pediatric

1. Introduction (definition of pediatric panic disorder)

- A panic attack is defined as an episode of intense fear, comprised of both physical symptoms (e.g. sweaty palms and heart pounding) and fearful thoughts (e.g. "I am going to die"). They usually last for about 10–15 minutes.

- Panic attacks are not caused by medical conditions or health problems and can occur any time.

- Panic attacks can occur in the context of many anxiety disorders (e.g. when someone with a needle phobia is about to get a shot); however, an individual may be diagnosed with panic disorder (PD) when they experience recurrent panic attacks that occur "out of the blue," resulting in intense anxiety between panic attacks about experiencing another panic attack and avoidance of situations in which panic attacks may be more likely to occur. Individuals with panic disorder commonly begin to experience symptoms in adolescence; panic disorder in younger children is less common [1].

1.1 The symptoms of panic disorder in children and teens

The children and adolescents with PD can experience the symptoms such as heart palpitations, difficulty breathing, sweating, hot or cold flashes, dizziness, trembling, numbness or tingling in the limbs, fear of dying or losing control, feeling as if one is in a dream, fear of going crazy, and sometimes feeling like one needs to "escape" during a panic attack. Cognition of these symptoms is very important, because parents and families can inform the pediatric psychiatry emergency for primary intervention [2].

Panic symptoms often can emerge quickly (within 10 minutes). Sometimes, the symptoms will be last for minutes or hours. Also, the children or teens may avoid from being alone or participating in kindergarten, schools, parks, or other places and need their caregivers or parents for leaving home [2].

1.2 Etiology, diagnosis, assessment and treatment

According to studies and researches, panic disorder etiology can be emerged by the biological, environmental, and social factors which can lead to disorder. For example, fear of animals, sexual or physical abuse, post traumatic stress disorder (PTSD), aggressive parents, problems in schools, high schools, and preschools, parent's divorce, and mental trauma can lead to panic disorder in children and teens [2]. For the most valid assessment in these children and teens, the Multidimensional Anxiety Scale for Children, the Screen for Child Anxiety and Related Emotional Disorders (SCARED), and the Spence Children's Anxiety Scale (SCAS) can be applied [3–5]. Sometimes, additional assessments as projective tests such as CAT, DAP (Drawing a Person), HTP (House-Tree-Person), DAF (Drawing a Family), and DAS (Drawing a School) may be useful. Because, drawing and paintings have projective elements in which we can see fears, anxiety, and stress in the form of drawing, size, colors, etc. [6, 7].

For treatment and psychological intervention, CBT (cognitive-behavioral therapy) and family education for control of the symptoms are the most common interventions and will be useful. Sometimes, medication may be necessary, especially in the acute cases [2].

2. Psychosocial problems and art therapy as a palliative and supportive intervention (family-based art therapy)

Psychosocial problems are highly prevalent among children and adolescents with an estimated prevalence of 10–20% worldwide [8, 9]. These problems can severely interfere with everyday functioning [10, 11].

Psychosocial problems in children and adolescents are a considerable expense to society and an important reason for using health care. But, most of all psychosocial problems can have a major impact on the future of the child's life [12]. For improvement of the psychological problems, especially anxiety, depression, and panic disorders, we can use cognition therapy, behavioral therapy, CBT, psychoanalytic intervention, and family counseling. But sometimes, one of the most important approaches in which children and teens with psychological problems can benefit is "Art Therapy" or AT [6, 7].

AT is one of the most important supportive-palliative interventions usually called family-based art therapy in which the children and adolescences can achieve their main abilities before their psychological problems, and also their families and parents participate in art therapy sessions actively [6, 13, 14]. Traditionally, AT is (among others) used to improve self-esteem and self-awareness, cultivate emotional resilience, enhance social skills, and reduce distress [15].

AT is a dynamic approach in which client and therapist create and will be created as soon as possible. In AT, the process in which changes are occurred will be more important and the art making result is less important, because all of the psychological changes will be occurred in the dynamic art process. Then, art therapist and art modalities such as painting, clay, crafts, and collage are the facilitators [16]. Also, art therapy approaches can be applied from infancy to adults, and the parents (in the most of cases "Mothers") have an important role in the art therapy process as a dynamic process in which the relationship between child and his or her parents will be reinforced [17, 18].

2.1 Art therapy approaches and the process relieve stress in panic and anxiety

We can explain the three art therapy approaches as follows: the humanistic art therapy, cognitive-behavioral art therapy, and expressive art therapy. All of these approaches are as palliative and supportive interventions which can be applied in the treatment of anxiety and panic attacks in children and adults. In the first approach which be called as the third force psychology, the clients are seen as a human not as a patient, because they are persons who suffer from a lot of problems such as anxiety and depression and the psychotherapists and art therapists have to support and help them by self-actualization. Josef Gary, an art therapist, has performed this approach according to three factors: 1. emphasis on solving the life problems, 2. encourage to self-actualization via creative expression, and 3. emphasis on self-esteem and attachment in the private relationships and social interaction and also survey for the life goals. Cognitive-behavioral art therapy is the second approach in which the cognition of the client will be changed via art therapy process, and finally he or she can achieve to self-actualization. And finally, in the third approach, art therapist can apply a large range of art modalities such as drama, dance/movement, music, and poetry/writing for the improvement of creativity in client and self-expression. Therefore, the third approach is called creative art therapy. The client's family and parents can involve in all of the art therapy approaches mentioned earlier. Therefore, we can call them as family-based art therapy intervention which can be applied for all the children and teens with psychological disorders such as panic, anxiety, and learning disorders and children with special needs. All of the mentioned art therapy approaches have common therapeutic objectives such as improvement of self-esteem, self-actualization, self-awareness, self-control, reinforcement of "ego," and projection of negative thoughts and feelings in children and teens via art works and activities [6, 13, 14].

Some of the art therapy techniques which can be applied for children and teens with panic and anxiety disorders are as follows: family painting, free association painting, collage, crafts, and clay. In all of these techniques, art therapist applies art modality instead of talking with client directly. Because, the children and teens can talk about their feelings by paintings and the other visual arts better than direct talking [14, 16]. **Figures 1–3** show the art works of clients who suffer from panic and anxiety. They have been referred, and both of them have participated in art therapy sessions along with their parents. Therefore, their art therapy sessions contained family-based art therapy program [6]. In all the techniques mentioned before such

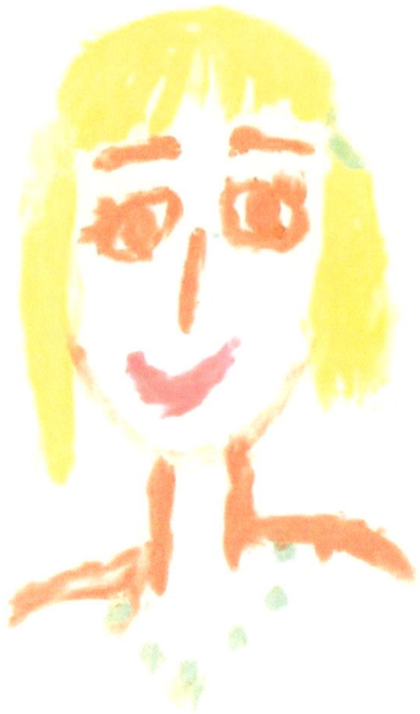

Figure 1.
Sheida, 9 years old girl, who illustrates her mother in her paintings.

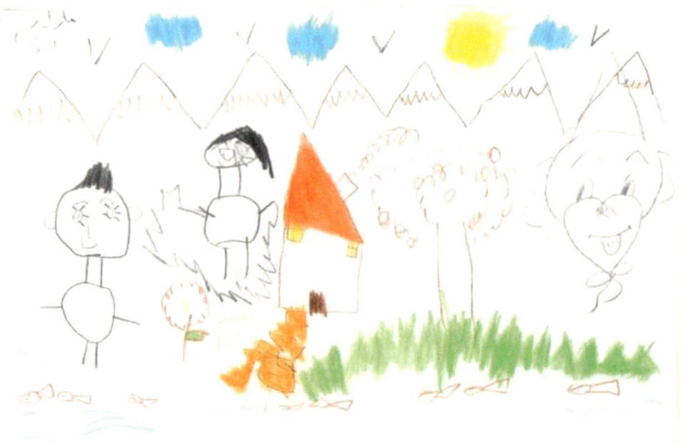

Figure 2.
Maziar, 17 years old boy, who illustrates fears and anxiety in his paintings.

as family painting, free association painting, collage, crafts, and clay, the therapist has focused on the client's changes during the art therapy sessions. They emphasize on therapeutic objectives such as improvement of self-esteem, self-actualization, self-awareness, self-control and reinforcement of "ego," and projection of negative thoughts and feelings in children and teens via art works and activities. Also, the client's family members and parents (especially mothers) are involved in the art therapy process actively [6, 7].

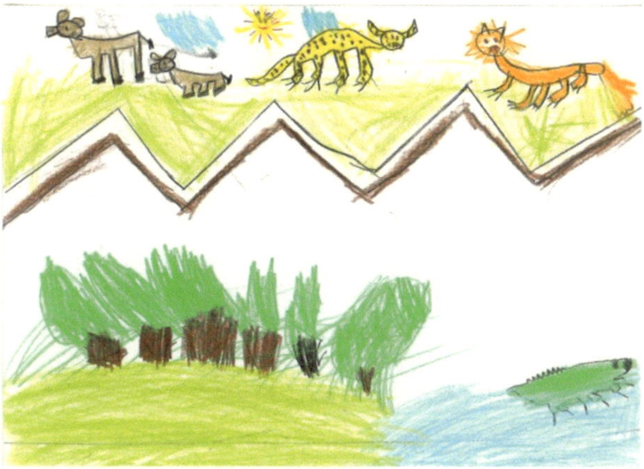

Figure 3.
Maziar and his fears.

Now the two case studies which have been investigated by the author are as follows:

Case study 1.

Sheida is a 9-year-old girl who suffers from panic disorder and has experienced anxiety since 2014. She had avoided from being in popular places, and withdrawal, anxiety, dizziness, trembling, numbness or tingling in the limbs, fear of dying or losing control, and feeling as if one is in a dream in this client could be observed. All of these symptoms caused secondary problems such as academic and family interaction problems. During art therapy sessions, creative art therapy was applied. She liked music and painting together. At first, she has been evaluated by projective psychological tests, and then family-based art therapy program was performed for her and her parents. Her mother had very important role in her tension release because she has applied family painting and free paintings and collage actively. They drew the fearful situations in their paintings and drawings and talked about their emotions together. The art therapist could facilitate the process of emotional release by talking about her paintings and help her in better cognition of ego. After five sessions, Sheida could overcome the loss of control and withdrawal. Also, she could participate in peer group activities such as painting and clay. Now, it seems that Sheida could show better self-esteem, self-control, and self-awareness and can control her anxiety by art making activities [6, 7].

Case study 2.

Maziar is a 17-year-old boy who lives with his parents, and he shows pathological phobia about animals like cat, dog, and birds. This kind of phobia leads to panic attacks, and he could not be calmed. He was resisting about attendance in park, streets, and crowded places without his parents and also showed obsession and stereotypical behaviors which disrupt his function. After necessary projective assessments, art therapy process special creative art therapy approach has been applied for him and his parents for 2 years. At first, he was illustrating fearful items like animals in his paintings, and then his parent (mother) involved in family-based art therapy program actively. He could talk about his fears and anxiety about animals step by step, and he could show better self-esteem and self-control while dealing with animals. Now, he has better self-esteem and shows interest in group plays with peers. **Figures 2** and **3** show his anxiety and fears [6, 7].

2.2 Literature review about art therapy and anxiety disorder

Some researchers have focused on the effectiveness of art therapy in anxiety and panic disorders such as Albertini who explain art therapy program in the treatment of agoraphobia and applying free paintings which can help clients for emotional expression [19], or Griffith who has explained brief cognitive-behavioral art therapy for anxiety disorders in her MS thesis. She has illustrated that art therapy can be useful in insight and cognition change in clients with panic and anxiety disorder. Indeed, she has applied cognitive-behavioral art therapy approach [20]. Also, Rosal has explained cognitive-behavioral art therapy in the research which can be useful for clients with anxiety [21]. Daneshmandi et al. have emphasized the effectiveness of family-based art therapy on children with generalized anxiety disorder (GAD) in their research [22]. Kheradmand et al. have investigated the effectiveness of art therapy on mental disorders such as anxiety and panic disorders in children [23]. Also, Hinz has investigated the effectiveness of art therapy assessment and treatment planning as an expressive therapy [24].

3. Conclusion

Panic disorder is one of the psychological disorders which can be observed in children and teens. Heart palpitations, difficulty breathing, sweating, hot or cold flashes, dizziness, trembling, numbness or tingling in the limbs, fear of dying or losing control, feeling as if one is in a dream, fear of going crazy, and sometimes feeling like one needs to "escape" are the symptoms which can be observed during panic attacks in children and teens.

For the assessment of these children and teens, the Multidimensional Anxiety Scale for Children, the Screen for Child Anxiety and Related Emotional Disorders (SCARED), and the Spence Children's Anxiety Scale (SCAS) can be applied. Not only CBT is one of the most common interventions which can be used for children and teens who suffer from panic disorder, but also art therapy as a palliative and supportive intervention can be useful for them. The common art mediums used within the art therapy process include painting, drawing, sculpture, collage, and photography. Three art therapy approaches are as follows: the humanistic art therapy, cognitive-behavioral art therapy, and expressive art therapy which all of them can be effective in panic and anxiety disorders. According to studies and researches, in art therapy process, art therapist can change the cognition, emotion, and behavior of the client by art modalities. Art therapy can be useful for children and teens too, because they can show their fears, anxiety, and emotions better than adults by paintings and other visual arts. Therefore, their paintings and drawings contain the meaningful messages which can be interpreted by the psychologist and art therapists. For the best outcomes of the art therapy, it can be followed by the children's family and parents at home as the family-based art therapy intervention. Finally, it is suggested that for the best anxiety and panic management, art therapy interventions are applied beside the other interventions such as play therapy, cognition therapy, and psychotherapy at clinics and schools.

A. Appendices

A.1 Anxiety

Art therapy
Art therapy process
Cognitive-behavioral art therapy
Expressive art therapy
Family-based art therapy
Humanistic art therapy
Self-expression
Self-awareness
Stress
Supportive and palliative interventions
Panic disorder

Author details

Kaveh Moghaddam
Exceptional Children Psychology and Art Therapist, Assistant Professor of Islamic Azad University, Tehran, Iran

*Address all correspondence to: kaveh_m_2000@yahoo.com; dockm1358@yahoo.com

References

[1] Andrew L, Hardy S, Saleh A, Ryee M, Willing L. Pediatric panic disorder. Available from: http://www.childrensnational.org. 2021

[2] Ganji M. Abnormal Psychology Based on DSM –V. 3rd ed. Tehran, Iran: Savalan Publication; 2021. pp. 707-710

[3] March JS, Parker JD, Sullivan K, Stallings P, Conners CK. The multidimensional anxiety scale for children (MASC): Factor structure, reliability, and validity. Journal of the American Academy of Child and Adolescent Psychiatry. 1997;**36**(4):554-565

[4] Birmaher B, Brent DA, Chiappetta L, Bridge J, Monga S, Baugher M. Psychometric properties of the screen for child anxiety related emotional disorders (SCARED): A replication study. Journal of the American Academy of Child and Adolescent Psychiatry. 1999;**38**(10):1230-1236

[5] Spence SH. A measure of anxiety symptoms among children. Behaviour Research and Therapy. 1998;**36**:545-566

[6] Moghaddam K. editor. Art Tehrapy and Anxiety. Workshop of the First Razavi International Anxiety Congress; Mashhad Iran; 2012

[7] Moghaddam K. editor. The role of painting and drawing on evaluation and treatment of anxiety in children. First Razavi International Anxiety Congress; Mashhad. Iran. 8-9 Oct 2012

[8] Kieling C, Baker-Henningham H, Belfer M, Conti G, Ertem I, Omigbodun O, et al. Child and adolescent mental health worldwide: Evidence for action. The Lancet. 2011;**378**(9801):1515-1525

[9] Child and adolescent mental health. World Health Organization. 2018 [cited 2018]

[10] Bhosale S, Singru S, Khismatrao D. Study of psychosocial problems among adolescent students in Pune, India. Al Ameen Journal of Medical Sciences. 2015;**8**(2):150-155

[11] Veldman K, Reijneveld SA, Ortiz JA, Verhulst FC, Bültmann U. Mental health trajectories from childhood to young adulthood affect the educational and employment status of young adults: Results from the TRAILS study. Journal of Epidemiology and Community Health. 2015;**69**(6):588-593

[12] Smith JP, Smith GC. Long-term economic costs of psychological problems during childhood. Social Science & Medicine. 2010;**71**(1):110-115

[13] Moghaddam K. Painting and Clay Therapy in Children and Adolescents with Autism Spectrum Disorder. Tehran. Iran: Narvan Publication; 2021. pp. 44-53

[14] Moghaddam K. Design and Effectiveness of the Family-based Art Therapy Program on the Marital Satisfaction of Parents,Verbal Skills, Social Interactions and Stereptypical Behaviors of the Autistic Children [Science and Research Branch]. Tehran: Islamic Azad University; 2015

[15] Facts, figures and helpful resources from AATA (American Art Therapy Association). Available from: https://multibriefs.com/briefs/aata/review122117.pdf2017

[16] Zadeh Mohammadi A. Art Therapy, an Introduction of Art Therapy Special for Groups. Tehran, Iran: Ghatreh Publication; 2010. pp. 18-20

[17] Case C, Dalley T. Art Therapy with Children From Infancy to Adolescence. USA & UK, Newyork & London: Routledge; 2008. pp. 20-24

[18] Case C, Dalley T. Working with Children in Art Therapy. 2nd ed. UK, London: Routledge; 2006. pp. 30-31

[19] Albertini C. Contribution of art therapy in the treatment of agoraphobia with panic disorder USA. American Journal of Art Therapy. 2001;**40**(2):137-147 Online ISSN:0007-4764

[20] Grifith FJ. Brief cognitive behavioral art therapy for anxiety disorders. [Thesis for MS] USA: Yale University; 2013.

[21] Rosal M. Cognitive behavioral art therapy, [Thesis in MS]. USA: Florida State University; 2001

[22] Danshmandi E, Jahan F. The effectiveness of family-centred art therapy on anxiety sensitivity, inefficient attitudes, and coping of students with generalizad anxiety disorder (GAD). Journal of Exceptional Children Empowerment. 2021;**12.4**(37):38-48. DOI: 10.22034/CECIRANJ.2021.259157.1525

[23] Kheradmand F, Abdollahin D, Mahmoodi R. The effectivenss of art therapy on mental disorders. Available from: http://Civilica.com/doc/778635 (OSConf 02-167)

[24] Hinz L. Enhancing art therapy assessment & treatment planning with the expressive therapies continuum. [Thesis]. USA: Dominican University of California; 2016

Chapter 4

Panic Disorder and Burnout in the Workplace: Review of the Evidence and Recommendations for Future Research

Olga Lainidi, Eva Tzioti, Maria Spiliou, Panagiota Koutsimani and Anthony Montgomery

Abstract

Both panic disorders and burnout are significant challenges in the workplace. However, to date knowledge in these areas has progressed in parallel and there have been few attempts to systematically connect these overlapping syndromes. The objectives of this chapter are to address this gap in the literature by addressing the following: how panic disorder symptoms can be masked under the "burnout-umbrella" meaning they can go under-the-radar, how the overlap between sub-clinical anxiety physical symptoms and panic disorder symptoms might lead to the latter remaining undiagnosed, and the extent to which burnout can contribute to experiencing panic disorder symptoms. Particularly, we will focus on professions that require high levels of emotional labor (e.g., healthcare employees, teaching professions) and which are characterized by pathological altruism, where individuals feel that they are not allowed to experience a panic attack in their work environment—and if they do, they will have to hide it. Moreover, such hiding leads to increased feelings of guilt and apathy, which in turn increases the likelihood of a depressive symptomatology to be developed. Finally, we argue that the field is hampered by the fact that employees are less likely to report the real intensity of their anxiety and stress-related symptoms.

Keywords: panic attack, burnout, anxiety, workplace stress, workplace well-being

1. Introduction

Panic disorder is a significant challenge in the workplace. Personal stories of experiencing a panic attack at work or because of work-related stressors can be easily found in anecdotal evidence, blogs, and informal conversations. However, the literature looking directly into the relationship between work stressors and panic disorder is scarce, and we believe does not reflect the real extent of the issue nor what work-related problems can be hidden behind employees' panic attacks. For example, the concept of "workplace phobia" (WP) – which from a clinical perspective is characterized by similar symptoms as agoraphobia – however, has had very limited research interest, as a quick search with no time restrictions on some of the main databases (e.g., Pub Med) yields only eight results with the words "workplace phobia" in their title. While WP incorporates psychophysiological symptoms that manifest upon exposure (*in vivo* or *in vitro*) to the workplace, it is considered to be mainly characterized by avoidant behaviors and there is insufficient evidence to consider how often it might manifest in the form of panic attacks [1, 2].

Asai et al. [3] explored the relationships between job stressors (e.g., job strain; effort reward imbalance; workplace social support) and panic attack/panic disorder in a Japanese working population. Panic attacks/disorders were measured by self-report. The results indicated that for the Japanese working population, high effort/reward imbalance is more likely to lead to PA/PD compared with low effort/reward imbalance. Of course, the clinical psychology literature has indicated cultural differences in the definitions and experiences of anxiety among different countries that might result from the differences in sociocultural norms, values, and expectations [4]. As such, findings on the subject might differ by different cultures/countries.

More is known about the prevalence of panic attacks among healthcare professional after the COVID-19 pandemic compared with either pre-pandemic times or other occupations. Alonso et al., [5] in their longitudinal study on the impact of COVID-19 on Spanish healthcare workers, measured probable current mental disorders including major depressive disorder (MDD), Generalized Anxiety Disorder (GAD), Post-Traumatic Stress Disorder (PTSD), and Substance Used Disorders (SUDs) and work-related factors (e.g., care center preparedness, weekly working hours) among other variables. Panic attacks were measured as the number of panic attacks experienced in the 30 days prior to the interview. The prevalence of Panic Attacks was 23.9% at baseline and 19.5% at 4-month follow-up; MDD, GAD, and PTSD followed a similar tendency, however, there was a slight increase in self-reported SUDs. Panic attacks have also been recently studied among teachers with evidence suggesting that teachers may suffer from panic attacks and anxiety and often feel alone and unsupported [6].

In the following sections, we identify some reasons behind the lack of clear evidence on the relationship between work stressors and panic attacks as well as potential ways that this kind of evidence could potentially help us understand better the literature around work stress and burnout.

2. Job Burnout and panic disorder: the missing links

2.1 Job Burnout

The increasing evidence on occupational burnout among different professional groups has highlighted that burnout is potentially a "human" aspect of work, meaning that all individuals might experience burnout symptoms at some point in their life in most occupations. While this book focuses on panic disorder, we believe that we cannot position panic disorder in the workplace well-being literature without discussing the relationship between burnout and anxiety. Though experiences of burnout have appeared across cultures and history for a very long time, the systematic study of burnout did not start until the 1970s, when Freudenberger [7] described occupational burnout for the first time, focusing on the experiences of weariness and/or exhaustion as a result of the work demands in one's occupation. Christina Maslach later defined burnout as a psychological syndrome that involves a prolonged response to chronic

DOI: http://dx.doi.org/10.5772/intechopen.107533

emotional and interpersonal stressors on the job [8]. The three key dimensions of job burnout are exhaustion, feelings of cynicism/depersonalization, and a sense of professional inefficacy/lack of accomplishment [9]. Exhaustion is the individual stress dimension of burnout, and it refers to feelings of being physically overextended and depleted of one's emotional resources; cynicism (or depersonalization) refers to a negative, callous, or excessively detached response to other people; and inefficacy (or lack of accomplishment) refers to a decline in one's feelings of competence and successful achievement in one's work [10].

There is significant debate over the "nature" of burnout; in a nutshell, some researchers support the conceptualization of burnout as a *psychological condition that reflects some disordered functioning in the individual*, and as such, should be approached as a psychological disorder [11]. Thus, we should advocate for solutions on the individual level. Other researchers, however, support that burnout is an *organizational problem* [12]; thus, we advocate for solutions on the organizational level. Over time, there have been several suggestions regarding burnout being the same as or an expression of *depression or/and anxiety or/and stress*. There is still some disagreement over the causes and mechanisms of job burnout, as not everyone gets burnt out by doing the same job in the same organization; it does not take the same time for all individuals to experience feelings of burnout; people respond to burnout differently; some professions might exacerbate either of the dimensions more or faster than others.

Despite the literature suggesting that burnout should be viewed as a psychological condition, it is not classified as a disorder by the American Psychiatric Association in their latest Diagnostic and Statistical Manual [13]. However, it has been added in the latest International Disease Classification (ICD-11) by the World Health Organization [14] as a "syndrome that results from chronic workplace stress that has not been successfully managed," providing the three dimensions of exhaustion, cynicism, and professional efficacy as its manifestation. As it is included in the section related to employment/unemployment, it has been suggested that the ICD-11 definition reflects an occupational phenomenon and not a medical condition, and as such the emphasis should be put on the work environment and the fact that job demands and resources are in a mismatch, thus not allowing the person to do their work in a meaningful and non-distressing way.

2.2 Burnout and panic disorder

As panic attack disorder is one of the anxiety disorders [13], in order to better understand the literature around panic disorder in the workplace, it is important that we first briefly discuss the relationship between job burnout and anxiety. To this end, both burnout and anxiety share a significant positive relationship with neuroticism [15]—a personality trait that indicates emotional instability and sensitivity to stress. Thus, the higher the neuroticism, the more likely that somebody will experience anxiety and/or burnout. Extroversion, on the other hand, has been found to have a negative relationship with burnout and with anxiety [15]; thus, the more extroverted someone is, the less likely it is for them to experience anxiety and/or burnout. Meta-analytic findings have also suggested that job burnout is a predictor of 12 somatic diseases, including coronary heart disease, headaches, respiratory diseases, and early mortality (before the age of 45 years old) [16]. This increases the need for further research on the extent to which stress-response mechanisms are in fact underlying burnout in a way similar to anxiety disorders. So, if the two actually share important physiological and psychological mechanisms, can job burnout exacerbate the experience of panic attacks? Can work contribute so much to anxiety that employees experience panic attacks in or out of the workplace?

The direct evidence linking job burnout and panic disorder is limited [17]. From a physiological point of view, burnout and panic disorder share common neural circuits as frontal and limbic brain structures appear to underlie both syndromes. Indeed, meta-analytic findings show that there is a significant relationship between burnout and anxiety [18] while there has been some evidence in favor of a common neurobiological basis. A systematic review regarding the potential impact of burnout on limbic brain structures has concluded that there is an impact in terms of HPA dysregulation (hypothalamus-pituitary-adrenal axis), impaired neurogenesis, and limbic structures atrophy; this could be an indication that stress is an integral part of burnout from a physiological perspective that could be further expressed in the form of a comorbid anxiety disorder, especially when no other measures are taken to relieve the stress caused by burnout [19].

Four key brain regions that are implicated in burnout and panic disorder are the prefrontal cortex (PFC), the cingulate cortex, the amygdala, and the hippocampus.

Burned-out employees and individuals suffering from panic attack disorder show deactivation of the prefrontal and cingulate cortex, reduced hippocampal activation, and an increased amygdala engagement [20–22]. The PFC is mainly responsible for executive functions such as inhibition, working memory, and decision-making; a set of cognitive functions that support goal-directed behavior and adaptive responses—thus, it is no surprise that a fundamental symptom of burnout and panic attack disorder is the sense of lack of control. The cingulate cortex is involved—among others—in the formation and processing of emotions; the hippocampus is a key area for learning and memory while the amygdala is mostly known about its role in emotional responses. Disconnection between the frontal and limbic brain regions results in behaviors and emotions common to burnout and panic attack disorder as well (e.g., lack of control, feeling of detachment, difficulty in regulating one's emotions), as well as to anxiety disorders generally.

These physiological responses are mediated by "bottom-up" and "top-down" processes. The "bottom-up" process, as the term suggests, involves the ventral nervous system; i.e., the amygdala and the hypothalamus. The amygdala is responsible for appraising and detecting threatening stimuli and regulates the hypothalamus, which, in turn, controls the neuroendocrine response toward the stressful stimulus [23]. The "top-down" (i.e., the dorsal nervous system) process includes the PFC and hippocampal brain regions. One major role of the PFC is to regulate the neuroendocrine response, the effects of the stress hormones in the amygdala and the hippocampus [24], and negative emotions [25]. In layman's terms, when the working environment cultivates stressful situations (e.g., strict deadlines, toxic supervisors/coworkers etc.), the bottom-up network perceives these situations as threats that need to be dealt with by fighting or fleeing. Prolonged activation of the bottom-up network leads to a dysregulation of the top-down network; thus, the individual is no longer able to evaluate and manage the environmental stimuli in a more rational manner. Meanwhile, extended stressful periods ultimately result in an under-activated top-down network that is unable to effectively assess the incoming environmental stimuli and hence, inhibit the over-activation of the bottom-up network. This process leads to a limited ability in appraising the (in)significance of the environmental stimuli; making the individual more vulnerable to the stressful situations they encounter in both their work and personal lives, and thus more susceptible in burnout and/or panic attacks.

All in all, this underlying common physiological mechanism not only indicates that the onset of one of the two disorders can exacerbate (or initiate) the symptoms of the other disorder, but also suggests that the distinction between the two syndromes based on a limited array of diagnostic techniques can be a tricky and difficult task. Neuroimaging techniques, for instance, are an essential diagnostic tool in the field of neuroscience as they aid experts to gain a better understanding of the neurobiological mechanisms responsible for the expression of a set of behaviors, assisting this way the differential diagnosis. All the same, one could argue that both burnout and panic disorder fall under the umbrella of stress, hence the common neurobiological background of the two syndromes and the likelihood of the two syndromes co-occurring come as no surprise. An observation that also raises the question if and in what way and degree burnout and panic attack disorder are differentiated from each other. Therefore, the shared mechanism between the two syndromes demands careful and detailed screening with the use of thorough clinical interviews for detecting burnout or panic disorder or a potential comorbidity of the two, if burnout is approached as a psychological disorder (based on the previously discussed debate on the nature of burnout). On the other hand, approaching burnout as an organizational problem allows considering the possibility of burnout being a cause of stress–and thus a cause of panic attacks. The context of one's thoughts, emotions, and behavior should be taken into consideration when assessing for psychological disorders that fall under the spectrum of anxiety. Indicatively, [17] reported a significant positive relationship between job burnout and panic disorders among nurses in Canada; nurses reporting higher burnout levels were 23 times more likely to screen positive for panic disorder while 20.3% of Canadian nurses were positively screened for panic disorder. However, the cross-sectional design of the study does not provide information regarding the causal linkages between the two syndromes. That is, are burned-out employees more sensitive to panic attacks; and if so, how burnout severity and duration affect the onset/duration of these panic attacks? Is there a specific burnout dimension that shows stronger associations with panic attack disorder? On the other hand, do individuals who have been diagnosed with panic attack disorder develop burnout more often compared with the individuals with no such diagnosis—perhaps, due to the emotional wear out that accompanies (frequent) panic attacks? We need to look further into the relationship between burnout and panic attack disorder.

The aforementioned ICD-11 classification [14] highlights that when "diagnosing" burnout, it is important to rule out any potential adjustment disorders; anxiety disorders and mood disorders (i.e., depression). Meanwhile, in the literature it remains unclear whether and to what extent burnout can be differentiated from anxiety or depression as well as whether burnout can "exist" without some level of anxiety and/or depressive symptoms, even of subclinical level. The activation of the HPA axis has also been linked to anticipatory anxiety, which in turn can increase the probability of a panic attack [26]. Research on the relationship between anxiety and job burnout, however, is not "anxiety-disorder" specific, in that research related to occupational health and workplace well-being mostly consists of self-reported measures of anxiety (e.g., HADS, STAI, etc.) [18], thus measuring the very common psychological condition of responding to stressors on a cognitive, emotional, behavioral, or physiological level in general, and the state/trait anxiety dimensions are usually not controlled for.

2.2.1 How can burnout be linked to panic disorder?

Though burnout seems to share variance with depression, anxiety and anxiety-related disorders [18, 19], existing evidence indicates that burnout and anxiety are not overlapping constructs [18]; this suggests that this is probably the case with burnout and panic disorder as well. As mentioned before, very little has been reported on the relationship between burnout and panic attacks, though we believe that further exploration of that relationship could help us better understand the nature of burnout and its relationship to anxiety. One of the main difficulties in burnout research is the inability to identify when somebody starts experiencing burnout symptoms, as these do not appear in an acute form and can build up over days, weeks, months, or years of exposure to a profession or a work environment or work-related stressors. Moreover, not all professionals in the same profession experience burnout working in different organizations and not all employees of the same organization experience burnout [27]—as burnout highly varies within and between individuals. We believe that exploring the relationship between burnout and panic attacks/disorder can provide some significant benefits that can shed more light on the burnout literature. For example, unlike burnout, panic attacks are "episodic," which means that it is probably easier for an employee to recall when they experienced their first panic attack compared with when they started experiencing burnout symptoms. The symptoms experienced during a panic attack are probably clearer and more agreed upon by clinicians and researchers (see chapter of this book on what is a panic attack) compared with those of burnout, which makes identifying burnout more challenging than diagnosing panic attacks. On many occasions, employees might not be aware that they have started to feel burnt out until the subjective experience of their work starts having a spillover effect on other aspects of their life (e.g., quality of sleep; health-related behaviors; interpersonal stress, depressed/cynical mood, etc.). However, it is more likely that they will start noticing physical symptoms of stress that might resemble to those of a panic attack, even if they have not experienced a complete panic attack yet—and not consider that experience as being necessarily work-driven. This might also contribute to our understanding of the burnout-anxiety-depression timeline as still it is not clear which comes first: anxiety, burnout, or depression; and whether these appear in some chronological order or as a vicious cycle with stress being in the center. For example, do entry-level employees experience physical stress symptoms more intensely than their senior counterparts, if the latter are emotionally exhausted and more cynical toward their job demands (i.e., higher burnout level)?

Obviously, the aforementioned relationships are more complicated than linear, direct effects, and we do not expect that one pathway might be sufficient to explain how the experience of panic attack symptoms relates to burnout or vice versa. To that end, we propose three initial pathways as potential starting points. These are merely suggestions and hypotheses aiming to drive an interest in the relationship between burnout and panic attack symptomatology.

The first pathway is related to the sense of control/autonomy that employees might experience in their work environment. Karasek 's [28] model of workplace stress—the demand-control model—suggests that while high job expectations are not inherently detrimental, they might cause stress if they are combined with little room for control. The importance of having a sense of control as a psychological resource is known to have stress-buffering effects in and out of the work-related literature. Many researchers have since corroborated these findings; when given greater job control, employees exhibit lower levels of anxiety and role overload, but when given less job control, employees exhibit higher levels of worry and a sense of role overload [29, 30]. Low or no sense of control over one's environment (work) can be a significant stressor that could possibly initiate a strong stress response leading to panic attack symptoms. This is expected to be more common among lower-ranking workers, who usually have a lot less control and autonomy. Interestingly, such a hypothesis was tested on non-primates, showing an interesting link between social rank and stress. In particular, studying baboons, Sapolsky [31] found that lower ranking individuals in a society of baboons that had less control due to their hierarchy, had also higher levels of cortisol, the stress hormone. Building on this rationale, a study from Harvard in 2022 [32] came to test these findings in the workplace, by researching the relationship between leaders, control, and stress. Up to that point being a leader had been portrayed as being extremely stressful in both the social scientific and practitioner literatures, as the higher rank one holds in their workplace, the higher the responsibilities—and the higher the expected levels of stress. However, research on leaders' physiology came to contradict that. Leaders have a unique psychological resource—a sense of control—that may act as a stress-reduction mechanism and was seen by their lower cortisol levels and self-reports on stress. To that end, further research into biomarkers of stress, experiences of panic attack symptoms, and screening for panic disorder among workers with low sense of control/autonomy is required to examine whether looking into physiological stress due to low control/autonomy will actually contribute to redesigning jobs and healthy workplaces for lower-ranking positions more effectively than diagnosing burnout has. What is more, cognitive neuroscience could also focus on the extent to which brain functioning and thus, cognitive functioning affect stress responses; e.g., do employees with low sense of control demonstrate by nature a "top-down" deactivation (and thus, lower executive function skills) and "bottom-up" over-activation?

The second pathway looks at work-related stress beyond "working in a stressful environment" but in fact as a source of "survival anxiety," since job security is critical for meeting the foundational physiological and psychological needs in order to survive. A recent study on the effects of income and job loss on mental health indicated that panic attacks are significantly more common among individuals experiencing income loss. de Miquel et al. [33] focused specifically on employees with job loss and income loss during the COVID-19 Pandemic indicating that approximately 11% of the participants had experienced at least one panic attack in the last 30 days and income loss was identified as a significant predictor of panic attacks with the highest odds ratio compared to depression and PTSD. The relationship between income loss and panic attacks remained significant in the model adjusting for age, gender, marital status, and educational level. For people experiencing income loss, the probability of experiencing at least one panic attack was 39% higher compared with individuals who did not experience an income loss. Panic attacks are, thus, a stress response to the uncertainty and insecurity caused by a work-related income loss; this highlights the overarching effect of work-related stressors as for a majority of people work-related income is crucial for survival, as perceived financial stress partially mediated the relationship between income loss and presence of panic attacks. This study highlighted that these work-related stressors are not only related to the work environment (e.g., toxic leadership, relationships with colleagues, etc.) but also to the realistic role that having a job plays in having an income that allows for meeting physiological and psychological needs. To that end, panic attack symptoms are expected to be more common among employees with low job security; minimum wage employees; employees who are at risk of job loss and/or income loss/reduction and could be ignored or misdiagnosed as burnout due to the emotional exhaustion or pessimist stance toward their work.

The third pathway is related to the aspects of emotional and personal involvement in one's profession through what is known as emotional labor. Emotional labor is based on the idea that employees are often forced to display emotions at odds with what they truly feel and is the result of the groundbreaking work of sociologist

Arlie Hochschild [34]. A good example for the understanding of emotional labor is the teaching profession. Being a teacher implies a considerable amount of personal involvement, availability, and constant interaction with others. Further occupational stressors may also be present, such as tremendous workloads [6] and imbalance between social and emotional demands [35]. Teachers who have higher job involvement are significantly more likely to develop anxiety disorder symptoms [36]. In addition, burnout symptoms are commonly developed among individuals in teaching positions; however, it is not something that is openly discussed due to the stigma around it. Maslach's three-dimensional model of burnout [8] applies for teaching positions as well, involving emotional exhaustion, depersonalization, reduced productivity, and decreased personal accomplishment. These represent great losses in the educational field for both teachers and learners. However, teachers are invited to control and regulate their emotional expressions in the classroom, and this involves tremendous effort for emotional suppression and regulation, which might lead to increased stress levels that could result in panic attacks. The latter might happen in the workplace or be "brought home"; in the latter case, it is less likely for the individual to identify the panic attack as work-related. Working as a teacher involves maintaining professionalism through all kinds of interactions, inside and outside the classroom. The pressure to remain constantly strong and emotionally available and the feeling of failure when this cannot be delivered have a great impact in teachers' well-being. Furthermore, it is very common that expressing emotional exhaustion, work overload, and burnout carries a big amount of guilt, as these are assumed to be part of the job. This might sometimes mean that teaching positions require plenty of personal time and dedication, which are frequently taken in the cost of private life. Most of these negative emotions and feelings, however, cannot not be displayed and experienced at work, where teachers are expected to display emotions that are aligned with their professional identity, leading a form of a dark cycle where burnout is symptomatic of anxiety and panic attacks, trying to remain professional in the classroom.

3. Are work-related panic attacks going under the radar?

The answer is YES—but it is difficult to demonstrate this via empirical research, and our supposition is corroborated by anecdotal evidence, informal conversations and "off the record" interviews, pop-psychology articles, and blog pieces. While there is an increasing research interest regarding the relationship between anxiety and workplace well-being and work-place stressors, the specificity of the scientific knowledge on the topic is significantly limited by (some) critical factors:

3.1 Research tools measuring anxiety "in general"—and not always!

Most of the literature looking into anxiety/stress in the workplace fails to report on experiences of physiological stress symptoms, including panic attack symptomatology. We will use the well-known Hospital Anxiety Depression Scale (HADS) [37] as an example to further explain. HADS is probably the most common tool used to measure anxiety in studies related to workplace well-being and anxiety in the workplace; meta-analytic findings suggest that studies that used the HADS reported stronger relationships between burnout and anxiety compared to studies that used other scales, while interestingly the relationship was slightly less strong among healthcare professional than in the general employed population. These limitations can be further highlighted by the fact that between 2013 and 2018, only one longitudinal study was identified on the relationship between anxiety and burnout [18].

HADS was designed to help measure anxiety symptoms in patient/hospital settings (e.g., patients with coronary heart disease), and there is no evidence of a latent variable structure, being frequently criticized for not being sensitive enough to differentiate between depression and anxiety as clearly as claimed [38]. A 10-year systematic review [38] revealed anomalous factor loadings of both anxiety and depression items on depression and anxiety respectively or on both factors. This suggests that some of the items included in the HADS do not represent clearly depressive or anxiety symptoms, as these could be potentially present in both cases. With regard to the experience of somatic symptoms that might be an indicator of anxiety or panic attacks, no somatic items had been included in the construction of this scale—mostly due to the fact that the scale was designed for hospital/patient samples, and thus, somatic symptoms are expected to be common due to health conditions (e.g., cardiovascular heart disease) [39]. The scale includes one item that reads "I get sudden feelings of panic" (answered on a four-point Likert scale), which, although at a face validity level seems relevant to panic disorder, the phrasing "feelings of panic" is up for interpretation by each participant; the word "panic" when used in daily life and not in clinical/psychological contexts might indicate excessive worry, intense fear or anxiety, feelings of helplessness, or "not knowing what to do," anticipation anxiety, distress (etc.). Thus, one of the most widely used measures for anxiety in studies looking into working populations does not have any references to somatic symptoms or the experience of panic attacks, as it has been developed to be administered to patient/hospital samples. In that case, if participants from working populations experience panic attacks or even somatic symptoms that can indicate panic-disorder risk, this is most likely to go under radar due to the instruments that are most commonly used in quantitative studies. In practical terms, this mean that if the employees of an organization are screened for anxiety with the use of the HADS, the screening results will not provide any information on whether any of the employees suffer or are at risk of suffering from panic attacks. Thus, despite the findings connecting work with anxiety—such as the relationship between anxiety and job burnout—the evidence on how/whether work contributes to panic attacks and/or panic disorders is rare and cannot be validly deduced from screening instruments such as the HADS.

3.2 A technocratic approach to anxiety among working populations: differentiating or compartmentalizing?

Measuring anxiety in working populations has almost become a "habit," especially when researchers include measures of burnout in their studies. Moreover, there are references to work-related anxiety [40]; job anxiety [41] or job-related anxiety, which is separated into team-job related anxiety and individual job-related anxiety [42]; employee anxiety[43]; to these we would also like to add other closely related concepts such as work stress [44]; work-related stress [45]; job-related stress [46]; job stress [47]; occupational stress [48]; organizational stress [49]. This is indicative of one of the well-recognized difficulties in conducting research related to stress and anxiety, as discrepancies in the operationalization and definition of the concepts are wide and very common, while each field and discipline is looking at stress and anxiety from different perspectives. There is no consensus as to whether stress and anxiety are independent variables (i.e., causes or contributing factors), whether they are outcomes (i.e., results from other causes and contributing factors), or whether they are mediating processes critical in understanding how work-related life impacts overall mental and physical health and general quality of life. Especially in the work-related literature, the almost nonexistent experimental studies along with the very few longitudinal studies with limited validity regarding causal models testing and the overwhelming number of cross-sectional studies have led to a reciprocal understanding of the relationship between the different types of work-related stressors and anxiety outcomes. In this difficult to navigate literature, the use of generic anxiety measures as explained before makes practical implications even more difficult to delineate, as although we know that during difficult times at work, working populations are more likely to report higher anxiety levels, our understanding of what type of anxiety symptoms they are experiencing, when and where those symptoms are more intense as well as their meaning-making process is extremely limited. In addition, although the compartmentalization of anxiety might make it easier for quantitative analysis, the proof that work anxiety is indeed a "distinct" construct that is mainly the result of work-related stressors is also mostly built on theoretical assumptions and cross-sectional data; and in the meantime, there is no proof that work-related anxiety cannot be reduced by improving out-of-work quality of life or is different to anxiety induced from a toxic family culture. Such an assumption suggests that "compartmentalizing" anxiety into types based on the sphere of life might have some practical benefits, but it could also lead to several potential methodological artifacts, especially given that work life is mostly explored without controlling for personal and family life variables when it comes to quantitative research. We are not in any way implying that work life cannot be the main source of anxiety in a person's life; our concerns are related to the potential biases stemming from quantitative research that might overlook individual (e.g., personality, predisposition etc.) and out-of-work factors (e.g., contextual and socio-cultural factors) that could be significant in explaining work related anxiety.

We should be careful not to throw the baby out with the bathwater; of course, the research on work and anxiety has produced significant findings and has highlighted that working populations are undergoing extreme amounts of anxiety and stress to meet work demands—and many times beyond what is necessary for the job to be done (e.g., working with toxic supervisors). The identification of work-related mental health challenges is a very important step in creating healthy workplaces, and the work of several scholars has served as a milestone in advancing our understanding of the real impact that work life has on people's mental health [50, 51]. We wonder, however, whether this approach has now limited practical implications mainly driven by the need to produce generalizable and representative findings that serve the methodological axioms of quantitative research, which sometimes might result in a metaphysical obsession with method [52] rather than with how to identify who needs support and how we can provide it better. And while there are several taxonomies and sub-definitions of stress and anxiety for working populations, very little has been reported in studies regarding how often, e.g., employees in different professions and industries experience panic attacks in the work environment or out of it, when are panic attacks more likely to happen (e.g., prior, during, or after the shift), what percentage of affected employees seek help, whether they share this information with supervisors and coworkers, whether panic attacks at work are exacerbated during work-related crises or times of personal difficulty (etc). The need to address this gap in the literature becomes even more evident considering the several blogs, pop-psychology articles, personal testimonies, and anecdotal evidence that panic attacks in the workplace or panic attacks triggered by work demands are in fact very common. Articles and blog pieces entitled "Managing a Panic Attack at Work"[1] "Managing your panic Disorder at Work [2] "I had a panic attack at work. This is what happened [3] "What to do when a Panic Attack hits at work [4] frequently include information transferred from general therapeutic protocols for anxiety and panic attacks (e.g., CBT; Mindfulness etc.) in the form of tips. One article, however, entitled "My stressful job is giving me panic attacks, but I feel guilty leaving [5] by Alison Greens, owner of the blog "Ask a Manager [6] can help further understand the complexity of dealing with panic attacks (e.g., CBT; Mindfulness etc.) in the form of tips. One article, however, entitled "My stressful job is giving me panic attacks, but I feel guilty leaving" by Alison Greens, owner of the blog "Ask a Manager" can help further understand the complexity of dealing with panic attacks at work or because of work, which goes beyond collecting data on the relationship between anxiety and burnout: employees and managers need support and help making sense out of the subjective experience of having a panic attack and what to do when it happens or when an employee informs them that they have been having panic attacks. The latter article highlights the guilt that employees might be experiencing when considering leaving a job that is potentially contributing to the decline of their mental and/or physical health, which in this case might also stem from a need for the employee to feel valuable and needed by their team and organization; e.g., "I cannot abandon my team because they need me"; "I feel guilty towards the manager who offered me the job," etc. Clinical literature supports that guilt is a key theme when it comes to mental health disorders [53], and literature on burnout has showcased that employees very often experience feelings of guilt as they cannot cope with the job demands due to insufficient resources (personal or organizational) [54]. And to that end, although compartmentalizing anxiety might help quantitative researchers, a multidisciplinary view of anxiety in the workplace might be more productive when looking into the experiences of the working populations.

3.3 "It's your fault you can't handle the pressure": panic attacks as "personal weakness" and the idolization of resilience

Work stress has been a major research topic especially with regard to healthcare professionals—not surprisingly so, as healthcare professionals rank among the top burnt-out work groups [55, 56]. All the available evidence points to the fact that the most healthcare systems in the world (e.g., the NHS in the UK) are under considerable stress. The overwhelming majority of healthcare workers wake up every day motivated to positively impact the patients they serve. Employees with a high calling intensity (such as healthcare professionals) are especially prone to the detrimental effects of emotionally disturbing work. The drive for healthcare employees, for example, to "keep going" and "get the job done" has a dark side referred to as pathological altruism, which refers to behaviors that attempt to promote the welfare of another but can have pernicious long-term consequences for the care giver [57].

---

1 https://hbr.org/2022/03/managing-a-panic-attack-at-work#:~:text=Common%20triggers%20at%20work%20include,Racing%20heart%20rate

2 https://www.verywellmind.com/panic-disorder-and-the-workplace-2584191

3 https://www.abc.net.au/everyday/i-had-a-panic-attack-at-work-this-is-what-happened/101115920

4 https://www.forbes.com/sites/stephaniesarkis/2019/11/21/what-to-do-when-a-panic-attack-hits-at-work/?sh=252b9b869427

5 https://www.thecut.com/article/my-job-started-giving-me-panic-attacks.html

6 https://www.askamanager.org/about

Such an approach very frequently idolizes resilience—in the sense of enduring hardship at any cost—to a degree that being able to handle any hardship, stress, and difficulties happening at or stemming from one's job becomes a badge of honor. Healthcare can exploit the professional ethic of healthcare professionals, which results in a form of dysfunctional professionalism that supports maladaptive healthcare structures in education and practice and which can influence staff at all levels.

We believe that this culture of "performance first" no matter the cost and the admiration of abnormally resilient employees has been transferred to many sectors and industries over time and has been further exacerbated by the economic crises, as these give permission to organizations and employers to use the "limited resources" narrative when imposing extreme demands on employees with non-equivalent benefits. The culture of "performance first" implies that showing any sign of difficulty to deal with work demands is a weakness and as such it is not "allowed." Personal stories from blogs include references to occasions when employees have managed to "press pause" on an upcoming anxiety or panic attack until they find themselves in a space where nobody can witness this "proof of personal weakness." A work culture like this adds more stress to an already stressful work life where, for example, meeting tight deadlines is one of the most valued attributes for corporate executives or managing to care for a disproportionate number of patients during a pandemic is one of the most valued attributes for nurses. Such cultures usually involve a non-speaking-up dimension as well, where employees feel that they are not actually allowed to express themselves and if they do so, this might have serious consequences. Therefore, symptoms of anxiety and panic disorder are more likely to be developed and usually left unattended. But the fact remains that having the "resilience" to endure the aforementioned along with several other stressors in both one's work and personal life has been an idolized profile for a very long time; this means that employees are less likely to openly communicate facing mental health difficulties, including experiencing panic attacks in or outside of work. Is it, then, any surprise that these highly motivated individuals feel numb or cynical toward interventions that seek to increase their "resilience" or "engagement"?

4. Recommendations and conclusions

Our knowledge about panic disorders in the workplace is significantly limited. This is an evidence gap when we consider the unclear field of coexisting and partially overlapping conditions that exists with the more frequently studied phenomena of burnout, stress, and anxiety. Moreover, a more fine-grained understanding of panic disorder and panic attacks in relation to work stressors might help better understand the role of the stress response mechanism in burnout.

This chapter has demonstrated that quantitative organizational researchers have ignored or overlooked the panic symptomatology in their use of generic scales (e.g., HADS) that purport to measure anxiety. We can speculate that panic disorders are more easily viewed as being under the remit of clinical psychology rather than that of occupational/organizational research. However, this is a missed opportunity as concepts such as rumination have been successfully imported from clinical psychology into occupational/organizational psychology. Additionally, panic disorders have the potential to help understand the nexus between work and non-work domains better, in that a panic disorder is more likely to be "brought home" in occupations with high levels of burnout.

DOI: http://dx.doi.org/10.5772/intechopen.107533

5. Summary of main points

Panic attacks are often described by psychologists as "attacks" taking place to notify the person that there is something wrong in their lives. Lack of control in one's life could be a reason a panic attack can occur—a red button alarm that is flashing and screams danger. The experience is acute and extremely uncomfortable as the person experiencing it thinks that death is near. The danger might not be "real"—they are not actually dying—but they might have a low control over their lives that is causing this overwhelming feeling of fear and lack of safety. If we could use a metaphor to describe it, the experience of stressful work can be like that of an animal facing grave danger but is locked in a cage and cannot act toward its safety. Work environments with low sense of psychological safety can resemble a cage, meaning that they limit the employees' ability for control and autonomy; this results in a sense of helplessness, which can lead to high stress levels and potentially panic attacks. The culture of stress and the strict hierarchies is common in most sectors and industries, with employees facing high demands, little control, and often a lack of empathy and attention to well-being. A closer focus on experiences of panic symptoms with the use of interviews (qualitative research) and scales measuring physiological stress symptoms/panic attack symptoms (quantitative research) will contribute to our understanding of how to create healthier workplaces.

Conflict of interest

The authors declare no conflict of interest.

Author details

Olga Lainidi[1*], Eva Tzioti[2], Maria Spiliou[3], Panagiota Koutsimani[4] and Anthony Montgomery[5]

1 University of Leeds, Leeds, UK

2 Mediterranean College, Thessaloniki, Greece

3 Aristotle University of Thessaloniki, Greece

4 University of Macedonia, Thessaloniki, Greece

5 Northumbria University, Newcastle, UK

*Address all correspondence to: lndolga@gmail.com

References

[1] Muschalla B, Linden M. ArbeitsplatzängsteundArbeitsplatzphobie und ihre Auswirkungen auf die berufliche Partizipation [Workplace-related anxiety, workplace phobia and disorders of participation]. Versicherungsmedizin German. PMID. 1 Jun 2009;**61**(2):63-68. 19544717

[2] Haines J, Williams CL, Carson JM. Workplace phobia: Psychological and psychophysiological mechanisms. International Journal of Stress Management. 2002;**9**(3):129-145. DOI: 1072-5245/02/0700-0129/0

[3] Asai Y, Imamura K, Kawakami N. Association of job stressors with panic attack and panic disorder in a working population in Japan: A cross-sectional study. Journal of Occupational and Environmental Medicine. 2017;**59**(6):516-521. DOI: 10.1097/JOM.0000000000001021

[4] Good BJ, Kleinman AM. Culture and anxiety: Cross-cultural evidence for the patterning of anxiety disorders. In: Tuma AH, Maser J, editors. NY: Routledge; 2019. pp. 297-324

[5] Alonso J, Vilagut G, Alayo I, Ferrer M, Amigo F, Aragón-Peña A, et al. Mental impact of Covid-19 among Spanish healthcare workers. In: A large longitudinal survey. Epidemiology and psychiatric sciences. 2022. p. 31

[6] Rasheed-Karim W. The influence of policy on emotional labour and burnout among further and adult education teachers in the U.K. International Journal of Emerging Technologies in Learning (iJET). 2020;**15**(24):232. DOI: 10.3991/ijet.v15i24.19307

[7] Freudenberger HJ. Staff burn-out. Journal of Social Issues. 1974;**30**:159-165. DOI: 10.1111/j.1540-4560.1974.tb00706.x

[8] Maslach C, Jackson SE, Leiter MP. Maslach Burnout Inventory. Manual. 3rd ed. Palo Alto, CA: Consulting Psychologists Press; 1996

[9] Leiter MP, Maslach C. Latent burnout profiles: A new approach to understanding the burnout experience. Burnout Research. 2016;**3**(4):89-100

[10] Montgomery A, Maslach C. Health care professionals'. In: Llewellyn CD, et al., editors. Cambridge Handbook of Psychology, Health and Medicine. Cambridge University Press; 2019;**353-356**

[11] Starrin B, Larsson G, Styrborn S. A review and critique of psychological approaches to the burn-out phenomenon. Scandinavian Journal of Caring Sciences. 1990;**4**(2):83-91

[12] MacKinnon M, Murray S. Reframing physician burnout as an organizational problem: A novel pragmatic approach to physician burnout. Academic Psychiatry. 2018;**42**(1):123-128

[13] American Psychiatric Association. Diagnostic and Statistical Manual of Mental Disorders. Fifth ed. Washington, DC: American Psychiatric Association; 2013

[14] World Health Organization. ICD-11 for Mortality and Morbidity Statistics 2018

[15] Middeldorp CM, Cath DC, Berg MVD, Beem AL, Dyck RV, Boomsma DI. The association of personality with anxious and depressive psychopathology. In: Canli T, editor. Biology of Personality and Individual

Differences. New York, NY: The Guilford Press; 2006. pp. 251-272

[16] Salvagioni DAJ, Melanda FN, Mesas AE, González AD, Gabani FL, de Andrade SM. Physical, psychological and occupational consequences of job burnout: A systematic review of prospective studies. PLoS One. 2017;**12**:e0185781. DOI: 10.1371/journal.pone.0185781

[17] Stelnicki AM et al. Associations between burnout and mental disorder symptoms among nurses in Canada. Canadian Journal of Nursing Research. 2021;**53**(3):254-263

[18] Koutsimani P, Montgomery A, Georganta K. The relationship between burnout, depression, and anxiety: A systematic review and meta-analysis. Frontiers in Psychology. 2019;**10**:284-302. DOI: 10.3389/fpsyg.2019.00284

[19] Bayes A, Tavella G, Parker G. The biology of burnout: Causes and consequences. The World Journal of Biological Psychiatry. 2021;**22**(9):686-698

[20] Durning SJ, Costanzo M, Artino AR Jr, Dyrbye LN, Beckman TJ, Schuwirth L, et al. Functional neuroimaging correlates of burnout among internal medicine residents and faculty members. Frontiers in Psychiatry. 2013;**4**:131

[21] Jovanovic H, Perski A, Berglund H, Savic I. Chronic stress is linked to 5-HT1A receptor changes and functional disintegration of the limbic networks. NeuroImage. 2011;**55**(3):1178-1188

[22] Perrotta G. Panic disorder: Definitions, contexts, neural correlates and clinical strategies. Current Trends in Clinical & Medical Sciences. 2019;**1**(2):1-10

[23] Kudielka BM, Kirschbaum C. Sex differences in HPA axis responses to stress: A review. Biological Psychology. 2005;**69**(1):113-132

[24] Maier SF, Amat J, Baratta MV, Paul E, Watkins LR. Behavioral control, the medial prefrontal cortex, and resilience. Dialogues in Clinical Neuroscience. 2006;**8**(4):397

[25] Savic I, Perski A, Osika W. MRI shows that exhaustion syndrome due to chronic occupational stress is associated with partially reversible cerebral changes. Cerebral Cortex. 2018;**28**(3):894-906

[26] Graeff FG, Zangrossi H Jr. The hypothalamic-pituitary-adrenal axis in anxiety and panic. Psychology & Neuroscience. 2010;**3**:3-8

[27] Bühler KE, Land T. Burnout and personality in intensive care: An empirical study. Hospital Topics. 2003;**81**:5-12. DOI: 10.1080/00185860309598028

[28] Karasek RA Jr. Job demands, job decision latitude, and mental strain: Implications for job redesign. Administrative Science Quarterly. 1979;**24**(2):285-308

[29] Taris TW et al. Job control and burnout across occupations. Psychological Reports. 2005;**97**(3):955-961

[30] Park H et al. Job control and burnout: A meta-analytic test of the conservation of resources model. Applied Psychology. 2014;**63**(4):607-642

[31] Sapolsky RM. The endocrine stress-response and social status in the wild baboon. Hormones and Behavior. 1982;**16**(3):279-292

[32] Sherman GD et al. Leadership is associated with lower levels of stress.

Proceedings of the National Academy of Sciences. 2012;**109**(44):17903-17907

[33] de Miquel C et al. The mental health of employees with job loss and income loss during the COVID-19 pandemic: The mediating role of perceived financial stress. International Journal of Environmental Research and Public Health. 2022;**19**(6):3158

[34] Hochschild AR. The Managed Heart: Commercialization of Human Feeling. Berkeley: Univ. Calif. Press; 1983

[35] Iancu AE, Rusu A, Măroiu C, Păcurar R, Maricuțoiu LP. The effectiveness of interventions aimed at reducing teacher burnout: A meta-analysis. Educational Psychology Review. 2017;**30**(2):373-396. DOI: 10.1007/s10648-017-9420-8

[36] Jones-Rincon A, Howard KJ. Anxiety in the workplace: A comprehensive occupational health evaluation of anxiety disorder in public school teachers. Journal of Applied Biobehavioral Research. 2018;**24**(1):e12133. DOI: 10.1111/jabr.12133

[37] Spinhoven PH et al. A validation study of the hospital anxiety and depression scale (HADS) in different groups of Dutch subjects. Psychological Medicine. 1997;**27**(2):363-370

[38] Cosco TD et al. Latent structure of the hospital anxiety and depression scale: A 10-year systematic review. Journal of Psychosomatic Research. 2012;**72**(3):180-184

[39] Coyne JC et al. Lack of prognostic value of type D personality for mortality in a large sample of heart failure patients. Psychosomatic Medicine. 2011;**73**(7):557-562

[40] Erickson SR et al. Severity of anxiety and work-related outcomes of patients with anxiety disorders. Depression and Anxiety. 2009;**26**(12):1165-1171

[41] Muschalla B, Linden M, Olbrich D. The relationship between job-anxiety and trait-anxiety—A differential diagnostic investigation with the job-anxiety-scale and the state-trait-anxiety-inventory. Journal of Anxiety Disorders. 2010;**24**(3):366-371

[42] Mao J et al. Team job-related anxiety and creativity: Investigating team-level and cross-level moderated curvilinear relationships. Journal of Organizational Behavior. 2021;**42**(1):34-47

[43] Ahmad A, Saud S. The effect of role overload on employee anxiety and organization citizenship behavior. Journal of Managerial Sciences. 2016;**10**:1

[44] Ganster DC, Rosen CC. Work stress and employee health: A multidisciplinary review. Journal of Management. 2013;**39**(5):1085-1122

[45] Rauschenbach C, et al. Age and work-related stress: A review and meta-analysis. Journal of Managerial Psychology. 2013;**28**(7/8):781-804

[46] Ratnawat RG, Jha PC. Impact of job related stress on employee performance: A review and research agenda. Journal of Business and Management. 2014;**16**(11):1-16

[47] LaMontagne AD et al. A systematic review of the job-stress intervention evaluation literature, 1990-2005. International Journal of Occupational and Environmental Health. 2007;**13**(3):268-280

[48] Singh C et al. Occupational stress facing nurse academics—A mixed-methods systematic review. Journal of Clinical Nursing. 2020;**29**(5-6):720-735

[49] Cooper CL, et al. Organizational stress: A review and critique of theory, research, and applications. Foundations for Organizational Science. Sage Publications. 2001

[50] Torquati L et al. Shift work and poor mental health: A meta-analysis of longitudinal studies. American Journal of Public Health. 2019;**109**(11):e13-e20

[51] Ford MT et al. Relationships between psychological, physical, and behavioural health and work performance: A review and meta-analysis. Work & Stress. 2011;**25**(3):185-204

[52] Robinson DN. An Intellectual History of Psychology. Wisconsin, USA: University of Wisconsin Press; 1995

[53] Carnì S et al. Intrapsychic and interpersonal guilt: A critical review of the recent literature. Cognitive Processing. 2013;**14**(4):333-346

[54] Gil-Monte PR. The influence of guilt on the relationship between burnout and depression. European Psychologist. 2012;**17**(3):231

[55] Benfante A et al. Traumatic stress in healthcare workers during COVID-19 pandemic: A review of the immediate impact. Frontiers in Psychology. 2020;**11**:2816

[56] d'Ettorre G et al. Post-traumatic stress symptoms in healthcare workers dealing with the COVID-19 pandemic: A systematic review. International Journal of Environmental Research and Public Health. 2021;**18**(2):601

[57] Wong AMF. Beyond burnout: Looking deeply into physician distress. Canadian Journal of Ophthalmology. 2020;**55**(3):7-16

Section 3

Interventions for Panic

Chapter 5

Psychotherapy of Panic Disorder: Revisiting Past and Present Research and Moving toward Future Directions

Behrooz Afshari

Abstract

Panic disorder is one of the most debilitating mental disorders. Therefore, it is necessary to apply treatments for this problem to eliminate the disability of patients. Both psychotherapy and medication have been shown to reduce the frequency and severity of panic attacks and panic disorder. In this chapter, we first mentioned cognitive-behavioral therapy as the cornerstone of psychotherapy for panic disorder and then, medication as one of the most common treatments for this disorder. Cognitive-behavioral therapy has been found by numerous studies to be the most important psychotherapy for panic attacks and panic disorder. Medication is another effective treatment because some medications can be very helpful in managing the symptoms of a panic attack as well as anxiety and depression. Finally, emotion regulation therapies for the treatment of panic disorder will be introduced and explained for the first time.

Keywords: panic disorder, cognitive-behavioral therapy, medication, emotion regulation therapies

1. Introduction

A severe acute attack of anxiety with a feeling of imminent harm is called panic disorder. People with panic disorder suffer from multiple panic attacks that are unrelated to specific situations. These attacks are periods of intense fear and physical discomfort; so the sick people feel that they cannot control themselves. The onset of these attacks is sudden and usually reaches its peak in 10 min. For a panic attack to be diagnosed as panic disorder, a person must have certain reactions to these attacks, including constant worry about the recurrence of attacks or worry about the consequences of the attacks, avoiding activities that may cause the physiological feelings associated with panic, or participation in safety-related behaviors, such as carrying a cell phone or medication [1]. Concerns about the consequences of attacks may include fear of having a fatal heart attack or fainting in front of others. Panic disorder is a unique disorder among anxiety disorders whose symptoms and signs are physical in the first stage. These patients are highly sensitive to unpredictable events, and their symptoms are almost related to one of three systems, including the autonomic nervous system (heart palpitations and sweating), the respiratory system (shortness of breath and chest tightness), and the cognitive system (personalization, fear of loss of control, and fear of death). This disorder is one of the most common disorders in the mental health system, so its prevalence is estimated at 5–9%. This disorder is associated with an increase in cardiovascular complications and mortality [2].

2. Investigating cognitive models of a panic attack

A panic attack is considered an acquired fear of bodily sensations (heart palpitations, dizziness, nausea, etc.), especially sensations associated with automatic arousal. In simple terms, after having panic attacks, people become over-sensitive to their physical feelings and feel threatened by any slight physical sensation and consider it as the possibility of starting a panic attack. Therefore, those who have panic disorder, after experiencing an unexpected panic attack, become anxious about experiencing such attacks in the future and are always worried about having these attacks again. Therefore, they become very sensitive to the smallest changes in their body to avoid panic attacks [3].

3. Why do we experience panic attacks?

From an evolutionary point of view, the reaction of fear or panic in the presence of a threatening situation is adaptive. It is assumed that panic occurs in the absence of a threatening stimulus, as a result of the interaction of stressful life events and psychological and biological vulnerabilities. The tendency to experience negative emotions, often labeled as neuroticism, is largely heritable and has been shown to predict panic attacks. This temperament probably acts as a biological vulnerability to experience fear (a rapid alarm response characterized by strong arousal of the nervous system) and experience anxiety (a negative mood state characterized by worry about future events and signs of physical tension) [4].

Environmental factors in childhood can play a key role in the formation of people's confidence and their abilities to control future life events. Such a sense of control or lack of control can act as a psychological vulnerability in the experience of fear and anxiety. Stressful life events, such as a new job or the death of a family member, may combine with biological and psychological vulnerabilities to trigger an emotional fear response or panic attack. Accumulated stressors built up over time by stressful life events can trigger a panic attack, even though the person perceives it as "unexpected" because there is no immediate threatening stimulus [5]. Therefore, three factors play a role in the occurrence of panic: (1) inheritance, (2) family environment in childhood, and (3) environmental factors.

4. After an unexpected panic attack, what causes the attacks to continue?

General vulnerabilities (heredity, family environment, and environmental factors) may play a key role in determining whether a person develops "anxious fear" about experiencing attacks in the future or not. In addition to general vulnerabilities in experiencing panic and anxiety, it is believed that there are specific vulnerabilities that contribute to the formation of panic attacks. An example is anxiety sensitivity. According to this belief, anxiety and its symptoms cause harmful physical, social, and psychological consequences beyond the physical discomfort of a panic attack. After a panic attack, a person becomes sensitive to the discovery of his bodily arousal, which leads to vulnerability to subsequent panic attacks [6].

Anxiety about unexpected panic attacks is linked to fear of physical sensations (such as heart racing) that accompany the attacks. At first, the person is anxious about their physical sensations and worries that it will lead to a panic attack. At this time, automatic thoughts such as catastrophizing (e.g., I will be ashamed if I have a panic attack) and over probability (e.g., If I go out I will have a panic attack) cause a person's anxiety to increase and as a result, physical feelings such as heart rate and dizziness increase. The increase in bodily sensations strengthens automatic thoughts and the person becomes more certain of the correctness of his beliefs, and as a result, these thoughts become stronger and cause more anxiety again. This self-perpetuating cycle continues until it results in a panic attack again [7].

5. Conditioning in a panic attack

Accompanying physical feelings with a panic attack makes a person more conditioned, and consequently becomes more sensitive to physical feelings. Then, physical feelings occur in all people sometimes and are resolved after a while; for a person with panic disorder, it means the beginning of a panic attack. Such anxiety about bodily sensations plays an essential role in the persistence of panic disorder. Physical sensations can be caused by physical activity, chemicals such as caffeine, a frightening environmental stimulus, and anxious images or thoughts. When physical sensations are noticed by a person suffering from panic disorder, they create fear. This fear intensifies bodily sensations and leads to an increase in that fear, and in turn, as a self-perpetuating cycle of fear and bodily sensations, leads to a further increase in bodily sensations, which ultimately leads to a panic attack. Therefore, the fear of experiencing physical sensations of arousal leads to a full-blown panic attack and reinforces the belief that these sensations should be feared [8].

To condition a person, it is sometimes enough to experience physical sensations with a panic attack once, and after that, other factors such as safety seeking and avoidance, which are explained below, cause the panic disorder to continue. People with panic disorder are often not aware that panic attacks can be triggered in this way (by bodily sensations or internal and external stimuli). For people with panic disorder, this means that panic attacks often occur unexpectedly and unpredictably. Because they cannot stop panic attack symptoms once they begin, they consider such attacks uncontrollable. The unpredictability and uncontrollability of a panic attack can fuel chronic anxiety levels, resulting in constant fear of another attack. Higher levels of chronic anxiety can lead to increased physical arousal as well as increased attention to one's bodily sensations. Increasing physical sensations and increasing attention to these sensations lead to an increase in the probability of panic attacks in the future [9].

6. How do avoidance and safety-seeking behaviors perpetuate panic attacks?

Behavioral responses to panic, especially safety-seeking behaviors (such as walking slowly to avoid elevated heart rate, not going to heights to avoid dizziness, and eating less food to prevent nausea) and avoidance (not leaving the house for fear of being attacked and avoiding lonely situations) apply as perpetuating factors of the panic disorder. A person with panic disorder mistakenly believes that a panic attack will cause catastrophic physical or mental harm, such as a heart attack, going crazy, passing out, or losing control. Therefore, experiencing panic attacks in which none of these things occur should necessarily undermine these beliefs [10].

However, people with panic disorder engage in certain safety-seeking behaviors that they believe enable them to escape or avoid the consequences of fear. For example, if a person believes they are going to pass out during a panic attack, they may sit or hold an object. Engaging in safety-seeking behaviors prevents a person from realizing that a panic attack does not cause a physical or psychological catastrophe because he believes that if he does not have a disaster, it is because he is sitting on a chair, or walking slowly, and not because a panic attack does not hurt him. Disconfirming false beliefs about panic attacks help to maintain the panic disorder. People may engage in safety-seeking behaviors designed to prevent panic or its feared consequences, such as taking antianxiety medication with them or traveling with people who make them feel safe [10].

Another behavioral response that perpetuates fear is overt avoidance. People tend to avoid certain places or situations that they believe are more likely to trigger a panic attack. Avoidance prevents the disconfirmation of false and catastrophic appraisals and reinforces the belief that these particular situations are dangerous, and increases the likelihood of having a panic attack in those situations in the future. Furthermore, if a person avoids situations in which they experienced an unexpected panic attack in the past, future attacks will inevitably spread to new, previously safe situations. Therefore, the range of safe conditions is limited. So most places become dangerous places where a panic attack is likely to occur. This pattern can increase behavioral avoidance and chronic levels of anxiety perception. Now let us look at useful techniques and therapies for treating panic disorder.

7. Psychological training in the treatment of the panic disorder

In the method of treating panic through psychoeducation, the therapist provides information to help correct the client's misconceptions about panic attacks and anxiety and to normalize the situation for him, which are effective for treating panic. In the first session of treatment, the therapist explains things about panic attacks so that these attacks become unpredictable and uncontrollable in the person's mind, and the person's misconceptions about panic symptoms, including the idea of going crazy, disappear, such as "When our ancestors were in the forests, they were residents, they were exposed to all kinds of natural disasters." Naturally, if they did not sleep at night with the fear of a lion or leopard attack, they would fall into such a deep sleep that they would not notice the presence of a lion or a leopard and become their prey [11]. Therefore, we are the descendants of ancestors who were worried about the dangers around them and were in a state of alertness.

8. The function of anxiety

The function of anxiety is to preserve the survival of the generation, and it is used when a person feels threatened. Now this danger can be real or imagined. At this time, anxiety is activated in the person's body and prepares him for fight or flight. That is, where it is possible to attack, attack the cause of fear, and otherwise, escape from the cause of fear. To prepare the body for fight or flight, changes are made in the body. Among other things, increasing the arousal of the autonomic nervous system, which controls many of our bodily processes, such as the cardiovascular and gastrointestinal systems. During anxiety, blood flow to the extremities of the body such as hands, feet, and arms increases, and blood flow to the head and internal organs decreases. Heart rate and breathing speed up and digestion slow down. These changes cause symptoms such as increased heart rate, shortness of breath, dizziness, and feelings of weakness and nausea. These symptoms all mean that the body is ready to face a dangerous factor, but it is not dangerous because they are used for the preservation and survival of the person and not to harm it. The problem arises when this survival protection system becomes overly sensitive, such as an over-sensitive burglar alarm that goes off at unnecessary and unhelpful times [12].

9. Cognitive factors in panic attacks

Another factor in panic attacks is the cognitive factor. The cognitive factor comes into action in the form of internal conversations: "Oh, what if my heart rate goes up? If I faint, my reputation will go down. I will have an attack at a party. How badly will they judge me if I have a panic attack? I'm going crazy." These negative thoughts intensify physical feelings. That is, they increase heart rate, intensify dizziness, and... The intensification of physical feelings, in turn, makes the person's negative thoughts stronger [13]. Also, he is more sure of the correctness of his belief that the attack will start. And he says to himself, "So I think I'm right that I'm having an attack." These symptoms are due to the negative cycle of physical feelings and negative thoughts that have intensified in the person. Finally, the arousal reaches the point where the person sometimes has an attack. As the number of these attacks increases, the person becomes more conditioned and more sensitive to his physical changes. He also noticed very small changes in his body and assumed it was a sign of the beginning of an attack.

10. Behavioral factors in panic attacks

Another factor in panic attacks is the behavioral factor. After the panic attack happened, the person adopts two strategies to deal with the risk of its recurrence [14], both of which cause the panic attack cycle to continue in the person: (1) Seeking safety and (2) avoid.

10.1 Seeking safety

In seeking safety, a person tries to reduce his sense of internal danger by using things that give him a sense of security. For example, wherever he goes, he takes his friend or his parents with him. In the case of each client, it should be investigated what factors he uses as safety so that after identifying its cases, little by little the client will face his imagined danger without them. In some cases, the use of sedatives is also considered a safety measure. Because the person thinks that these drugs have reduced his anxiety. Therefore, it is necessary to make exposure after some time when stopping the drug so that the person feels confident about himself [15].

10.2 Avoidance

In avoidance, a person avoids being in places or situations where he believes that the probability of a panic attack is high. This makes him never understand that these situations are not dangerous. Rather, the assumption is strengthened that if he was not attacked, it is because he avoided these situations [16]. The problem is that avoidance does not remain in one area and is constantly expanding. First, the lonely person is afraid of being attacked outside the city. He tells himself that in order not to be attacked, it is better not to go too far from the city. If he does what he thinks and avoids, the internal conversations become more threatening and this time he tells him not to be attacked from somewhere in the city. After some time, his inner dialog tells him again not to have a panic attack at a distance of more than 1 km from home. Finally, he reaches a stage where he cannot leave the house. Because he believed that it was his avoidance and seeking safety that caused him not to have a panic attack. In this case, it should be said that what helps a person treat panic without drugs is facing the issue of anxiety [17].

After being taught the three important components of fear and anxiety—physical symptoms, thoughts (cognitions), and behavior—as well as how they interact to contribute to panic disorder survival, clients are encouraged to list physical symptoms, thoughts, and behaviors related to their most recent episode of panic, and find out how their responses may prolong or exacerbate panic attacks. For example, when Tina realizes that her heart rate is fast, she is overcome with fear and has a panic attack, and faints. This alarming thought leads to a faster heart rate and other physical signs of anxiety, which ultimately increases his fear of having a panic attack. His behavior (rushing home, where it is safe) reinforces his belief that anywhere else is unsafe. Treatment aims to break this negative cycle by addressing the three main components of anxiety: changing self-talk or beliefs, controlling physiological responses, and confronting objects, situations, and places that cause fear [18].

11. Self-monitoring in the treatment of panic attack disease

In the treatment of panic attacks, the self-monitoring method helps the patients to observe their emotional reactions as an external observer instead of judging them subjectively. Self-monitoring can reduce anxiety, increase awareness of emotional reactions, and increase feelings of control [19]. For example, Tina's mental appraisal "I feel anxious, so there is no way I can go shopping" could be objectively described as "My heart beats faster. I think that if I go to the store, I will have a panic attack and faint." Clients are asked to complete a monitoring form for a recent panic attack that includes the following details: physical sensations, thoughts and behavioral reactions, the situation in which the attack occurred, and the degree of fear.

12. Teaching relaxation techniques in the treatment of panic

Breathing retraining is introduced as an adaptive skill in stopping physiological overreactions in the treatment of panic. The mechanisms by which breathing retraining is effective and the extent to which it is effective for panic are still under investigation. However, therapists must not use it as a means of avoiding negative emotions. The client is taught diaphragmatic breathing: breathing from the belly instead of the chest. The client is supposed to focus on his breathing by counting breaths (one) and thinking of the word "relaxation" as he exhales. For the first week of training, the therapist should breathe at a normal rate and speed. After 3–5 min of practice in the session, the client is assigned a breathing retraining task for the next week: 10 minu of practice, twice a day in a comfortable and quiet place [20].

13. Cognitive restructuring in the treatment of panic

Cognitive restructuring is the process of displacing automatic anxious thoughts or cognitive errors, such as risk overestimation and catastrophizing. In this case, therapists are taught how to identify their automatic anxious thoughts. Then, they are taught how to treat these thoughts as hypotheses and gather evidence to support or disprove them. Finally, they are encouraged to develop alternative hypotheses and gather evidence to support and reject them. Clients are explained that although anxious thoughts can be "automatic" and occur very quickly without full awareness, they can influence feelings and actions. The content of these thoughts is specific and may be different in different situations and times. Subsequently, it is important to identify or predict the specific content that creates anxiety in certain situations [21].

14. The "down arrow" technique for identifying automatic thoughts

Subjects are taught to use the "down arrow" technique to identify these automatic thoughts. The technique works like this: therapists ask themselves, for example, what they fear in a hypothetical situation. Then, they figure out what those fears would mean and what would happen if they were real. Then, the meaning of the thoughts of the lower layers is examined, and this process continues until the central anxious automatic thought is identified [22].

For example, Tina writes on her monitoring form: While driving, she became frightened when her heart rate increased. So she left the car and her mother sat behind the wheel instead. To uncover her automatic thinking, the therapist should ask her what would happen if her heart continued to beat. The therapist responds to Tina saying, "That is horrible!" she can ask what she imagines is happening that she finds terrifying. Again, in response to Tina saying, "My heart would beat faster, I would start shaking, and I would pass out," the therapist can ask what she thinks would happen if she experienced those feelings. The therapist can continue these questions until she gets to the central belief of her anxiety. The belief is that if she did not move the car, she would faint, have an accident, and kill herself and her mother. It is explained that identifying automatic thought is the first step in cognitive restructuring. And it should be practiced as part of this week's self-assessment assignment [23].

Then, they teach the audience to view their thoughts not as absolute facts, but as hypotheses. The Socratic questioning method is used to help them gather evidence to determine a more realistic possibility. For example, Tina thinks that the probability of losing control of the car and crashing during a panic attack is close to 100%. She is asked if this has happened before. Do you have any proof of its occurrence or nonoccurrence? After arriving at a more realistic possibility, the referent is assisted in generating alternative thoughts. For Tina, the alternative hypothesis might be: I'm just experiencing anxiety, and I'm also able to drive while experiencing anxious thoughts and bodily sensations [23].

15. Exposure in the treatment of panic

Repeated exposure to fearful physical feelings (physical exposure) and fearful situations (exposure in natural situations) to reject the incorrect cognitive evaluation and turn off conditioned emotional reactions to these feelings and situations is considered one of the main methods of panic treatment [24]. Using breathing retraining and cognitive restructuring to deal with these feelings and situations provides corrective experiences to therapists, which are not achieved by avoiding or running away from these feelings and fearful situations [24].

15.1 Exposure based on emotional arousal

First, physical exposure is done to increase learning about bodily sensations. Clients are told that their anxiety-provoking physical sensations are stimulated. To learn that these feelings are not harmful and can be tolerated. They remind them of the conditioning of bodily sensations and how minor changes in physiology can trigger anxious thoughts and physiological over-arousal in them due to prior pairing of bodily sensations with a panic attack [25].

Clients are reminded that avoiding changes in physical state or avoiding activities that cause changes in physical state (such as avoiding running because it raises the heart rate and evokes a panic attack) prevents remedial learning. Learning that physical symptoms are not harmful and can be tolerated. It is explained that avoidance perpetuates fear. By facing uncomfortable bodily sensations, they learn not to fear them [26].

Clients are directed to perform activities (e.g., climbing stairs, turning, gasping, etc.) to reexperience the bodily sensations experienced during a panic attack. They should continue the activity for 30 s after they first notice their bodily sensations. Then, record the bodily sensations they had, their level of anxiety, and how similar these sensations were to the bodily sensations experienced during the panic attack. An activity with a moderate degree of fear and little resemblance to the actual feelings of a panic attack is used to practice exposure to physical feelings within sessions and is assigned as a task (to be practiced three times a day) [27].

Clients are taught how to control the exercises by arousing emotions, assessing fear levels, using breathing retraining, and cognitive restructuring of adaptive skills [28]. Clients should answer these questions in each exercise: Did the disaster they feared (e.g., loss of control) happen? Did they survive from being scared? Did their fear subside with repetition?

15.2 Exposure to the natural environment

The next type of exposure is exposure in the natural environment: exposure in places and situations that clients avoid or fear. For the assignment, therapists must arrange a hierarchy of these situations by rating the intensity of the fear of each situation. A driving hierarchy for Tina (with fear rates in parentheses) might look like this: (1) Sitting in the car, (2) one-mile drive with mother in the car, (3) driving to the local store with mother, (4) five miles driving on the highway with mother, (5) driving to the local store alone, and (6) five miles of highway driving alone [29].

Subsequent sessions are devoted to safety cues, which include specific people and objects that make a person feel safe from anxiety, loss of control, physical injury, or embarrassment. In Tina's case, her house, her parents, and her inhaler were all signs of safety. Clients were explained that the removal of safety cues would improve the learning effect of the exposure [29]. When faced with situations with safety cues, the client still believes that the situations are dangerous, but the danger is prevented by safety signs. Abandoning safety cues are combined with direct exposure hierarchies [29].

16. Medication in the treatment of panic

Medication is one of the most popular and effective treatment options for panic disorder, panic attacks, and agoraphobia. Doctors may prescribe medication to reduce the severity of panic attacks, reduce overall feelings of anxiety, and potentially treat co-morbid conditions such as depression. Panic disorder medications usually fall into one of two categories: antidepressants and antianxiety medications.

17. Antidepressants for panic

Antidepressants are now commonly used to treat many anxiety disorders, including panic disorder and agoraphobia. Antidepressants affect the brain's chemical messengers known as neurotransmitters. It is thought that different types of these chemical messengers communicate between brain cells.

18. Types of antidepressants for panic disorder

18.1 Selective serotonin reuptake inhibitors

Selective serotonin reuptake inhibitors (SSRIs) are a popular class of antidepressants prescribed to reduce symptoms of anxiety and depression. Serotonin is a natural neurotransmitter in the brain. Studies have shown the long-term effects of SSRIs. These drugs have also been found to cause limited side effects, making them the prescription drugs of choice for panic disorder.

18.2 Tricyclic antidepressants

Since the introduction of SSRIs, tricyclic antidepressants (TCAs) have become less popular in the treatment of anxiety and mood disorders. However, TCAs are still an effective treatment option for people with anxiety disorders, including panic disorders. Like SSRIs, TCAs work by blocking the reuptake of the chemical messenger serotonin. In addition, many TCAs inhibit the reuptake of norepinephrine, another neurotransmitter in the brain that is often associated with the fight-or-flight stress response.

18.3 Monoamine oxidase inhibitors

Monoamine oxidase inhibitors (MAOIs) are one of the first antidepressants developed to effectively treat mood and anxiety disorders. MAOIs work by inhibiting the activity of the enzyme monoamine oxidase. This enzyme is involved in breaking down neurotransmitters, such as norepinephrine, serotonin, and dopamine. Dopamine helps to regulate many functions, including movement, physical energy levels, and feelings of motivation. Despite their effectiveness, MAOIs are used because of the dietary restrictions necessary and the potential for significant drug interactions that can occur when taking MAOIs with other medications.

18.4 Antianxiety drugs for panic

Antianxiety medications are prescribed to quickly relieve panic symptoms. These drugs work to calm the central nervous system, which can reduce the severity of panic attacks and make the person feel relaxed. Because of their sedative effect and quick relief, antianxiety drugs are often prescribed to treat panic disorder.

18.5 Benzodiazepines

Benzodiazepines are the most common class of antianxiety medications prescribed for panic disorder. Known for their sedative effect, these drugs can quickly reduce panic attack symptoms and induce a more relaxed state. By targeting gamma-aminobutyric acid (GABA) receptors in the brain, benzodiazepines slow down the central nervous system and induce a sense of relaxation. Despite the potential risks and side effects of these drugs, benzodiazepines provide safe and effective treatment.

18.6 Effective psychotherapies for panic disorder

18.6.1 Cognitive-behavioral therapy

Cognitive-behavioral therapy (CBT) in patients with mental disorders was initially developed to provide additional treatments for residual symptoms based on the principles and strategies of intervention previously developed for anxiety and depression. About 1% of psychiatric patients with persistent positive and negative symptoms do not need medication, even if they are compatible with prescription medications. However, despite the introduction of unusual antipsychotics, patient compliance with the drug is still a major problem. Studies have shown that 4% of outpatient and inpatient patients have stopped their treatment [30].

CBT in mental disorders is currently recognized as an effective intervention for mental disorders in clinical guidelines. Despite available evidence that side effects are absent, public access to this treatment in the community remains limited and low [31]. CBT is a goal-based approach to solving the problem of mental illness, especially mental disorders, to change the patterns of thinking or behavior that are behind people's problems and change their feelings. CBT in mental disorders is a common type of speech therapy (psychotherapy). You talk to a psychologist or psychotherapist in a structured way and with a specific number of sessions. This will help you identify the wrong or negative thinking so you can see the challenging situations more clearly and respond more effectively. CBT can be a very useful tool in the treatment of mental disorders, such as schizophrenia, depression, post-traumatic stress disorder, or an eating disorder, but not everyone who benefits from CBT in schizophrenic patients may necessarily have complete mental health. This therapy can be an effective tool to help anyone learn how to manage stressful life situations [32].

18.7 The benefits of CBT in mental disorders

CBT in mental disorders patients can also be effective in treating some mental health problems, but may not be effective for everyone. Some of the benefits of CBT in mental disorders include [32]:

- It may be helpful in cases where the drug alone does not work.
- Completes in a relatively shorter period than other speech therapies.
- The highly organized nature of CBT in mental disorders means it can be presented in a variety of formats, including in groups, tutorials, and computer programs.
- It teaches you useful and practical strategies that can be used in everyday life, even after treatment is completed.

The stages of CBT in mental disorders [33] usually include the following:

- Identify difficult situations in your life. These conditions may include medical conditions, divorce, sadness, anger, or symptoms of mental illness. You and your therapist may take some time to decide what goals you want to focus on.
- Know your thoughts, feelings, and beliefs about these problems. Once you have identified the problems you want to work on, your doctor will encourage you to share your thoughts about them. This sharing of thoughts may include talking to yourself about an experience, your interpretation of a situation, and your beliefs about yourself, your surroundings, and events. Your therapist may suggest that you record your thoughts.
- Identify negative or false thoughts. To help identify patterns of thinking and behavior that may help solve the problem, your doctor may ask you to consider your physical, emotional, and behavioral responses in different situations.
- Change negative or negative thoughts. The therapist encourages you to ask yourself whether your view of a situation is based on reality or a misunderstanding of what is happening! This step may be difficult for you because you probably need to spend a lot of time thinking about your life and yourself. Useful patterns of thought and behavior can become a habit with a practice that does not require much effort to use.

18.7.1 Treatment duration

CBT in mental disorders is generally a short-term therapy requiring approximately two to four sessions. You and your therapist can talk about the number of sessions that are right for you. Factors affecting the number of treatment sessions are as follows:

- Type of disorder or condition.
- Severity of symptoms.

- The length of time a person has had symptoms and spent with this condition.
- Speed up one's progress.
- The amount of stress the patient has.
- How much support do you get from family members and other people?

In general, CBT in mental disorders is of low risk. As this treatment usually relieves the patient's painful feelings and experiences, in some cases the person may feel unwell. You may be upset, crying, angry, or maybe physically weak during a challenging meeting. Some types of cognitive-behavioral therapy in mental disorders, such as the exposure phase, may put you in a situation where you have always wanted to escape. For example, if you are afraid of flying, you may be asked to board a plane. This situation can lead to temporary stress or anxiety. However, working with a skilled expert minimizes any risks. The coping skills you learn can help you manage and overcome negative emotions and fears [33].

Studies have shown that the results of short-term CBT continue for a long time after treatment. The effectiveness of cognitive therapies has been proven for most anxiety disorders. All kinds of psychological treatments are suggested to effectively deal with this disorder and also to deal with the problems caused by medication, but what should be considered is the difference between these interventions in terms of ease of implementation and continuity of treatment results. The treatment of muscle relaxation plays an important role in the new treatments of anxiety disorders. In research, Conrad and Ruth showed the effectiveness of relaxation therapy for anxiety disorders (generalized anxiety disorder and panic disorder). CBT is one of the basic treatments for panic disorder. In a study by Salkovskis and Warwick [34], the effectiveness of CBT on panic disorder was investigated. The results of this study showed that this treatment is very effective and the rate of recurrence of attacks after the implementation of this treatment method is insignificant.

18.8 Dialectal behavior therapy

Dialectical behavioral therapy (DBT) is a form of cognitive-behavioral therapy (CBT) that consists of a set of different techniques and treatments. These two treatments are technically different. DBT uses different languages, in addition to acceptance and mindfulness techniques. DBT considers judgment beyond CBT and is a way for clients to think, but it is not intended to change the way they think. Instead, the DBT acknowledges that there is a problem with how clients think, but the therapist first encourages clients to accept it instead of judging it and then helps them to do what they want. They can change, and look to make their thinking more balanced [35].

Although DBT was primarily designed to treat BPD, research has shown that it is helpful for other disorders [36–39]. We now know that this type of treatment is helpful for people who have difficulty adjusting their emotions, even if the cause is not related to a mental disorder. Due to the success of DBT in helping people learn to manage their emotions more effectively, today this treatment is increasingly being pursued by mental health professionals. Given the number of people seeking this form of treatment to help with their problems, there are unfortunately very few therapists who have been prominently trained in DBT.

18.9 DBT patterns

As mentioned earlier, the DBT model is made up of four components. Although DBT can be effectively presented to clients without these components, most research on BDT for BPD focuses on the whole pattern, which includes group skills training, individual therapy, telephone counseling, and counseling.

18.10 Group treatment

Group skills training is a structured and psychological group form of training designed to grow and increase clients' abilities. The group is formed once a week and is divided into four patterns: basic mindfulness skills, interpersonal effectiveness skills, emotion regulation skills, and distress tolerance skills.

18.10.1 Mindfulness skills

Linehan et al. [40] divided mindfulness skills into smaller sections to make it easier for clients to understand and integrate with their lives. The goal of mindfulness in treating disorders is to increase self-awareness. Increasing self-awareness helps clients become aware of their thoughts, motivations, and emotions and gradually learn to control them in more effective ways. Through mindfulness, clients also learn to tolerate thoughts, emotions, and motivations that they cannot tolerate and that they do not need to disclose their inner experiences, but can easily accept. Until these experiences gradually disappear.

18.10.2 Interpersonal effectiveness skills

The goal of these skills is to help clients reduce the interpersonal turmoil that often occurs in their lives and is basically about how to be more determined. Clients are taught to think about something that will allow them to make an acceptable interaction, and then they will learn techniques that will make them more likely to achieve this goal.

18.10.3 Emotion regulation skills

The goal of these skills is to reduce mood instability. Clients are taught general information about emotions, such as why we need them, and why we do not want to get rid of them even when they are completely painful. Clients learn the connection between their thoughts, feelings, and behaviors, and that changing one can affect the other. Self-validation through other techniques helps clients manage their emotions more effectively.

18.10.4 Disturbance tolerance skills

These skills are also known as "crisis survival" skills and aim to help clients without resorting to problematic behaviors, such as suicide attempts, self-harm, and substance abuse, to make something worse, to survive the crisis. These skills help clients stay calm and distract themselves from problems.

Group skills training as opposed to individual therapy for a variety of reasons: First, clients with problems with emotion regulation often go from one crisis to another, and when clients seek help because of this crisis, techniques training in an individual meeting is very difficult. In addition, an important aspect of any group meeting is credibility, for example, clients gain the experience of being in a group where others have a similar problem. Another advantage of the group is that the learning experience can be richer, such as when each client learns to follow the experience of other members. Finally, because interpersonal issues often arise in a group, this can be a great way to practice the techniques learned, as well as allow clients to learn how the technique works, use them more effectively, and get guidance [41].

18.11 Individual treatment

Clients usually attend one-on-one sessions with a DBT therapist once a week. The purpose of individual sessions is to help clients apply the skills learned in the group to reduce harmful behaviors, such as suicide, self-harm, drug use, and more. Like group meetings, individual meetings have a very clear shape and structure that will be discussed in detail in the following sections.

18.12 Telephone consultation

Telephone counseling is done to guide clients to use their skills. Telephone counseling means a brief interaction to help clients identify which techniques may be more helpful in the situation they are facing. It helps them overcome the barriers to using these skills and act more effectively.

18.13 Counseling team

According to Linehan et al. [40], DBT is meaningless without a counseling team. The structure of the DBT counseling team will vary depending on the therapist's environment. The team usually includes all DBT therapists in the clinic, such as social workers, psychologists, psychiatrists, and anyone working in individual therapy and skills training groups with DBT clients. For therapists who work privately, this is a little more complicated. Because teamwork is important in pursuing practice, private therapists may want to create a team that includes other private DBT therapists in their environment or even online, provided they adhere to it in secret. It does not have to be a big team. Depending on your situation, the team is used in two ways: First, to provide support to therapists and help them continue to develop techniques for working with clients using the DBT model, and second, to discuss the case. During the case study, the team assists the therapist to ensure that DBT techniques and strategies are adhered to. The team also feels exhausted and ineffective. In counseling sessions, the team uses DBT techniques such as taking a dialectical and nonjudgmental stance to prevent team members from engaging in power struggles and other dynamics that can disrupt the team and the healing process.

19. Effects of DBT on psychiatric disorders

Much research has been done on the use of DBT to treat other disorders besides BPD. Due to the large volume of research, only a summary of them is provided here, which is given below:

Researchers	Participants	Findings
Afshari and Hasani [37]	GAD patients	DBT helped to promote emotion regulation and mindfulness skills in the treatment of generalized anxiety disorder.
Afshari et al. [42]	Bipolar patients	DBT helped to promote executive function, emotion regulation, and mindfulness skills in the treatment of bipolar disorder.
Harley et al. [43]	treatment-resistant depressive patients	DBT leads to a significant improvement in treatment-resistant depressive patients.
Goldstein et al. [44]	Bipolar patients	DBT helps treat bipolar disorder in adolescents, and DBT techniques are also helpful in treating bipolar disorder in adults.
Nelson-Gray et al. [45]	Oppositional defiant disorder	Teaching DBT techniques to improve adolescent behavior with disobedience has been confrontational, practical, and promising.
Keuthen et al. [46]	Trichotillomania	The treatment for relapsing–remitting DBT has been a promising adaptation for obsessive–compulsive disorder (trichotillomania) with steady improvements over a six-month follow-up period.
Steil et al. [47]	PTSD	The DBT adapted for the post-traumatic stress disorder (PTSD) treatment related to sexual abuse in childhood has shown that the approach is promising.
Perepletchikova et al. [48]	Self-destructive behaviors	DBT was adapted to treat children who used self-destructive behaviors without suicide, with significant increases in coping skills and significant reductions in depression and suicidal ideation.
Rajalin et al. [49]	Family members of people with suicide attempts	The results showed a significant reduction in care responsibility, improved emotional health, and increased satisfaction with the patient.

Many specialists today are using DBT to treat illnesses and problems unrelated to the axis of a mental disorder. For example, Evershed et al. [50] used DBT to treat anger in male court patients and found that DBT had more benefits than patients who received conventional treatment. Sakdalan, Shaw, and Collier [51] found that DBT reduced the risk of suicidal ideation in patients with mental disabilities, and Drossell et al. [52] found that DBT First-degree caregivers of dementia patients helped to increase their search for appropriate behaviors, improved their psychosocial adjustment, increased their ability to cope, improved their emotional well-being, and reduced caregiver fatigue.

19.1 Stages of treatment

Linehan et al. [40] proposed a set of steps by which clients progress toward recovery: The direction of commitment and commitment (before treatment), the achievement of basic capacities (step 1), the reduction of post-traumatic stress (step 2), and increasing self-esteem and achievable goals (Step 3). In the rest of this section, we will summarize all the steps of Linehan.

19.2 Emotion regulation therapy

Emotion regulation therapy (ERT) is a manualized treatment that integrates components of cognitive-behavioral therapy, acceptance and commitment therapy, dialectical behavior therapy, mindfulness-based stress reduction, and emotion-focused treatments using a mechanistic framework drawn from basic and translational findings [37].

The goals of ERT are as follows:

1. Identifying, differentiating, and describing emotions, even in their most intense forms;

2. Increasing acceptance of affective experience;

3. Decreasing the use of emotional avoidance strategies (such as worry, rumination, and self-criticism);

4. Increase ability to utilize emotional information in identifying needs, making decisions, guiding thinking, motivating behavior, and managing interpersonal relationships and other contextual demands.

These skills are taught in the first half of the treatment and are then utilized by patients in an exposure/behavioral activation phase in the second half of the treatment.

19.3 Mindfulness-based cognitive therapy

Mindfulness-based cognitive therapy (MBCT) is a treatment protocol comprising meditation practices and cognitive behavior therapy skills. This treatment, which was formulated for unipolar depression, was later adapted for other psychiatric disorders [53].

Kabat-Zinn [54] argues that by adding mindfulness to the cognitive approach, it is easier to accept what has happened to the individual. The goal of mindfulness is to equip patients with ways to respond to life's stresses so that they can get rid of the psychological reactions that often exacerbate stress and interfere with effective problem-solving methods. Mindfulness therapy progressed rapidly to reduce stress. In this method, patients were taught to monitor their thoughts with a broader perspective and to have a decentralized relationship with their mental content. In the mindfulness method, what matters is how you feel free to understand that most thoughts are just thoughts and not objects or realities [55]. The simple act of recognizing thoughts as it can free the patient from the distorted reality often gives the patient more insight and a greater sense of control over life. Sometime later, the mindfulness model emerged based on the initial view of Kabat-Zinn [54] on treatment.

Mindfulness-based cognitive therapy is a new promise in explaining the cognitive-behavioral therapy approach. Mindfulness training requires metacognitive learning and new behavioral strategies to focus on attention, prevent mental ruminants, tend to worry, and expand new thoughts and reduce unpleasant emotions.

Mindfulness-based cognitive therapy (MBCT) is a combination of meditation, yoga, and cognitive therapy exercises developed by Segal et al. [53] to alleviate and treat human suffering, especially the emotional suffering of people. Expands to prepare for depression.

Mindfulness-based cognitive therapy is based on the Kabat-Zinn Mindfulness Stress Reduction Model, and the principles of cognitive therapy are added to it. This type of cognitive therapy includes various meditations, stretching yoga, basic training on depression, body review exercises, and several cognitive therapy exercises that show the relationship between mood, thoughts, feelings, and physical sensations. All of these exercises provide some sort of attention to physical and surrounding situations in the "present moment" and reduce automatic depressurization processes.

Mindfulness-based cognitive therapy is mind-based therapy and is one of the third-wave therapies [56]. In this style, the principles of cognitive therapy integrate with the mindset of mindfulness to improve emotional well-being and mental health.

19.4 Mindfulness-based stress reduction

According to the mindfulness-based stress reduction (MBSR) developed by John Kabat-Zinn, the main goal of the MBSR is to help people to improve their relationships with their thoughts, feelings, and physical feelings [57].

The MBSR was first practiced at the University of Massachusetts by John Kabat Zinn. In his stress-relieving clinic, participants were taught to practice mental relaxation with mindfulness. These efforts led to the formation of a mindfulness model based on stress reduction.

Currently, the most common method of mindfulness is MBSR, formerly known as the stress reduction program as well as relaxation. This method was designed in the structure of behavioral medicine and for a wide range of people with stress-related disorders and chronic pain. The program runs as an 8–10-week program for groups of more than 30 participants. In addition, meetings are held weekly and each session lasts about 2 h. Meeting instructions include practicing meditation skills, discussing stress, coping techniques, and homework.

Body examination, for example, is an exercise in which participants lie on the floor with their eyes closed for about 45 min, focusing their attention on different parts of their body, and carefully observing the emotions associated with each area of their body [58].

How mindfulness can act so markedly on resilience is still being studied, but it is now evident that the practice of mindfulness, if well learned, trains certain critical skills and changes the neurophysiology of the brain.

Furthermore, the MBSR is a practice-based, interactive learning program. Research shows the MBSR to be an effective complement to a wide variety of medical and psychological conditions. These include anxiety, asthma, cancer, chronic pain, depression, diabetes, fibromyalgia, gastrointestinal disorders, heart disease, hypertension, mood disorders, sleep disturbances, and stress disorders.

Mindfulness is the practice of *present-moment awareness.* It promotes personal well-being and enables us to experience life more fully by developing the ability to return with kindness to the present moment rather than being lost in repetitive thoughts and worries about the past or the future. In this way, we can make wise choices, rather than react unconsciously.

Becoming more aware of our thoughts, feelings, and sensations, in a way that suspends judgment and self-criticism, can have surprising results. Many people report finding inner strengths and resources that help them make wiser decisions about their health and life in general.

Most of us find ourselves "swept away" at times by a current of thoughts, feelings, worries, pressures, and responsibilities. We want things to be different from how they are right now. Feeling stuck in this way can be draining. Mindfulness can help us work directly with the struggle we sometimes have in relating to life's experiences. In doing so, we can greatly improve the quality of our life.

The MBSR is now taught in every state in the U.S. and in more than 30 countries. MBSR classes include instruction in mindfulness meditation, mindful movement, and other mindfulness practices, all guided by a skilled tutor.

For the program to be effective, your commitment to 45 minu of daily practice and active participation in all classes as well as the daylong retreat is important. The 8-week course meets for 2.5 h weekly. The all-day silent retreat provides an opportunity for participants to experience more deeply the mindfulness techniques learned in class.

Mindfulness means paying attention on purpose, nonjudgmentally, to what is happening in the present moment, both internally (physical sensations, thoughts, and emotions) and externally (sounds, sights, and smells). Mindfulness enables us to be in the present moment and aware of our experiences. This allows us to make more purposeful and wise choices, instead of reacting automatically (often with adverse consequences) to things we cannot control. Mindfulness also involves an intention to reduce or relieve suffering through the cultivation of kindness and compassion for oneself and others [59].

MBSR is appropriate for people with a wide variety of conditions, needs, and goals, including:

- Medical conditions such as cancer, chronic pain or fatigue, heart disease, diabetes, arthritis, seizures, autoimmune disorders, and many others;

- Psychological conditions including depression, anxiety, and sleep disorders;

- Stress in the context of work, relationships, school, finances, moving, and other situations;

- Illness prevention and wellness, cultivating balance in one's life, and developing a more consistent meditation practice;

- Health care providers, including physicians, nurses, pharmacists, physical therapists, mental health professionals, and others.

MBSR provides systematic training in both formal and informal ways to bring mindfulness into daily life. Formal practices, taught in class, include:

- The "body scan," in which participants systematically move their attention from head to toe;

- Sitting meditation, involving awareness of breathing, sounds, sights, thoughts, and emotions;

- Gentle movement (derived from Hatha yoga) and mindful walking, attending to physical sensations generated during movement;

- Loving-kindness meditation, a practice to help cultivate compassion for oneself and others.

Participants will also learn about the physiology of stress and how to use mindfulness skills in diverse contexts, including relationships, work, daily self-care, and managing physical symptoms. A central feature of this course is that participants are asked to engage in 45 minu of daily home practice, using recordings available on the web, as well as informal practice assignments, bringing mindfulness to daily activities they are already doing.

DOI: http://dx.doi.org/10.5772/intechopen.107482

19.5 Acceptance and commitment therapy

Acceptance and commitment therapy (ACT) was established by Hayes et al. [60]. This method is part of the third wave of behavioral therapies and followed by the second wave of these therapies such as cognitive-behavioral therapy. The ACT is affiliated with a research program called Communication System Theory. This approach accepts the change of thoughts and feelings instead of their transformation, content, or abundance [61]. This treatment is one of the most recently developed models whose key therapeutic processes are different from cognitive-behavioral therapy.

Its underlying principles include:

1. Accepting or wanting to experience pain or other disturbing events without trying to control them;

2. Value-based action or commitment combined with the desire to act as meaningful personal goals before the removal of unwanted experiences. Linguistic methods and cognitive processes interact with other nonverbal dependencies in a way that leads to healthy functioning. This approach includes practice-based exercises, language metaphors, and methods such as mental care [62].

The ACT is a model derived from the third wave of therapeutic behavior. The main goal of this model is to perform an effective action, an action that is conscious with full presence of mind and is value-oriented [61]. This model differs from traditional cognitive-behavioral therapy, which seeks to teach people almost how to control thoughts, feelings, memories, and other events, so it helps therapists with a sublime sense of self (spectator self). In general, in the third wave of therapeutic therapy, the main emphasis is on awareness of emotions and thoughts. In the ACT, the goal of the therapist is to increase psychological flexibility in clients. Accordingly, psychological flexibility means being able to go back to the present moment, be aware of and observe one's thoughts and emotions, distance oneself from rigid beliefs, and do what is important, despite unpleasant events [63].

The ACT derives its name from its two main messages: acceptance of what is beyond your control and commitment to an action that improves your living conditions and purpose. It is to maximize man's potential for a rich, fulfilling, and meaningful life. This is based on three main methods, which are as follows:

- Be present.

Consider yourself here and now, so you can react to life instantly and effectively.

- Welcome.

You will learn to change your relationship with these painful experiences, without drowning in them and instead of trying in vain to control them.

- Commit to important activities.

Identify what matters to you (we do not value it) and then use that knowledge to guide, inspire, and motivate you to change and improve your life [64].

Acceptance and occupational therapy also look at people in a health-oriented manner, so they are opposed to clinical diagnoses and base their work on a case-by-case *formulation*. In other words, the ACT refers to the two hexagons of psychological flexibility and nonpsychological flexibility. According to this model, those attending counseling or psychotherapy sessions are trapped in a hexagonal psychological inflexibility hexagon and suffer from an unreasonable conflict. Instead of communicating with the present, these people become captivated by mental rumination (past) and anxiety (future). In this case, the person experiences an avoidance (doing something to get rid of painful internal experiences that reduce a person's quality of life), intermingling (clinging to thoughts, judgments, or emotions), self-conceptualized attachment (effect verbal meaning that a person has created for himself or others), persistent inactivity (performing impulsive or passive behaviors or insisting on avoiding an experience that does not lead to a step in the direction of one's values), and not specifying values (lack of awareness of central values self or noncontact with them). Therefore, the main goal of the ACT is to live rich and valuable. The six aspects of psychological flexibility included: (1) contact with the present moment, (2) acceptance, (3) fault, (4) communication, (5) the definition of values, and (6) the committed action [65].

19.6 Metacognitive therapy

In the field of newer psychological treatments, metacognitive therapy was first introduced by Adrienne Wells. The term metacognition refers to cognitive processes that play a role in controlling different aspects of cognition. Although, based on many kinds of research, it can be concluded that psychological treatments have longer-term therapeutic effects than drug therapy alone on patients suffering from phobias, more efficient, shorter, and more accessible types of psychological treatments should be used as well. Metacognitive therapy was invented to improve the results of cognitive therapies. The effectiveness of behavioral-metacognitive therapy on mental disorders has also been confirmed. Wells and King [66] have proven the effectiveness of this treatment on generalized anxiety disorder, obsessive–compulsive disorder, and post-traumatic stress disorder, respectively. Studies show that anxiety disorders, including generalized anxiety disorder, respond to cognitive-behavioral therapy, but Wells, as the main creator of metacognitive therapies, believes that anxiety disorders, including generalized anxiety disorder, respond only to a certain extent to cognitive-behavioral therapy. What is emphasized in metacognitive therapy are factors that control thinking and change the state of mind, not challenges with thoughts and cognitive errors or long-term and repeated exposure to beliefs about trauma or physical symptoms [33].

20. Conclusion

This chapter outlined the most effective evidence-based psychotherapies for panic disorder, namely medication, cognitive behavior therapy, dialectical behavior therapy, mindfulness-based cognitive therapy, mindfulness-based stress reduction, acceptance and commitment therapy, and metacognitive therapy. Evidence suggests that medication may have an effect on the reduction of physical sensations associated with anxiety. However, cognitive behavior therapy is the common psychotherapy that addresses dysfunctional thinking and behavior in order to alleviate psychological problems in panic. The main technique in psychotherapy of panic disorder is exposure, which is significantly effective in treating panic. Other psychotherapies are not effective than cognitive behavior therapy and exposure.

Author details

Behrooz Afshari
Department of Clinical Psychology, Kashan University of Medical Sciences and Health Services, Kashan, Iran

*Address all correspondence to: behrooz.afshari71@gmail.com

References

[1] Baroni M, Frumento S, Cesari V, Gemignani A, Menicucci D, Rutigliano G. Unconscious processing of subliminal stimuli in panic disorder: A systematic review and meta-analysis. Neuroscience & Biobehavioral Reviews. 2021;**128**:136-151

[2] Bang M, Kim B, Lee KS, Choi TK, Lee S-H. Effectiveness of mindfulness-based cognitive therapy for positive clinical outcome in panic disorder: A 5-year longitudinal study. Mindfulness. 2021;**12**(9):2149-2160

[3] Hewitt OM, Tomlin A, Waite P. The experience of panic attacks in adolescents: An interpretative phenomenological analysis study. Emotional and Behavioural Difficulties. 2021;**26**(3):240-253

[4] Chalmers KJ, Rossetto A, Reavley NJ, Jorm AF, Kitchener BA, Kelly CM, et al. Redevelopment of mental health first aid guidelines for supporting someone experiencing a panic attack: A Delphi study. BMC Psychology. 2022;**10**(1):1-11

[5] Kamata K, Maruyama T, Komatsu R, Ozaki M. Intraoperative panic attack in patients undergoing awake craniotomy: A retrospective analysis of risk factors. Journal of Anesthesia. 2021;**35**(6):854-861

[6] Paal E. Eight seconds of panic. Narrative Inquiry in Bioethics. 2021;**11**(1):63-65

[7] Herjanto H, Amin M, Purington EF. Panic buying: The effect of thinking style and situational ambiguity. Journal of Retailing and Consumer Services. 2021;**60**:102455

[8] Chystovska YY. Panic disorders as somatic and neurotic states of personality: Conditioning, behavioural learning. Fundamental and Applied Researches in Practice of Leading Scientific Schools. 2021;**43**(1):49-54

[9] Morriss J, Zuj DV, Mertens G. The role of intolerance of uncertainty in classical threat conditioning: Recent developments and directions for future research. International Journal of Psychophysiology. 2021;**166**:116-126

[10] Kannis-Dymand L, Grace E, McDonald L, Chambers R. Australian and New Zealand psychologists' perceptions and use of therapist-guided exposure for panic disorder. Clinical Psychologist. 2022;**26**(1):11-22

[11] Shin B, Oh J, Kim B-H, Kim HE, Kim H, Kim S, et al. Effectiveness of self-guided virtual reality–based cognitive behavioral therapy for panic disorder: Randomized controlled trial. JMIR Mental Health. 2021;**8**(11):e30590

[12] Kenwood MM, Kalin NH, Barbas H. The prefrontal cortex, pathological anxiety, and anxiety disorders. Neuropsychopharmacology. 2022;**47**(1):260-275

[13] Smith NS, Bauer BW, Capron DW. Comparing symptom networks of daytime and nocturnal panic attacks in a community-based sample. Journal of Anxiety Disorders. 2022;**85**:102514

[14] Kılıç HS, Alkar ÖY. Predicting factors of cognitive Behavioral therapy process and outcome for panic disorder: An overview of mechanisms of change. Journal of Cognitive-Behavioral Psychotherapy and Research. 2021;**10**(3):315-315

[15] Clark AE, Goodwin SR, Marks RM, Belcher AM, Heinlein E, Bennett ME, et al. A narrative literature review of the epidemiology, etiology, and treatment of

co-occurring panic disorder and opioid use disorder. Journal of Dual Diagnosis. 2021;**17**(4):313-332

[16] Curtiss JE, Levine DS, Rosenbaum JF, Baker A. Cognitive-behavioral strategies to manage panic disorder. Psychiatric Annals. 2021;**51**(5):216-220

[17] Stephens A, Collette B, Hidalgo-Munoz A, Fort A, Evennou M, Jallais C. The quiet passenger: Cognitions, avoidance, and onset among people with driving anxiety. Transportation Research Part F: Traffic Psychology and Behaviour. 2022;**87**:30-41

[18] Richter J, Pietzner A, Koenig J, Thayer JF, Pané-Farré CA, Gerlach AL, et al. Vagal control of the heart decreases during increasing imminence of interoceptive threat in patients with panic disorder and agoraphobia. Scientific Reports. 2021;**11**(1):1-12

[19] Choi JY, George M, Yun SY. Development of a smartphone application for Korean patients with chronic obstructive pulmonary disease: Self-monitoring based action plans. Applied Nursing Research. 2021;**61**:151475

[20] Clouston T. Applied Relaxation. Payne's Handbook of Relaxation Techniques E-Book: A Practical Handbook for the Health Care Professional. 2021. p. 107

[21] Purdon C. Cognitive Restructuring. 2021

[22] Kürümlüoğlugil R, Tanrıverdi D. The effects of the psychoeducation on cognitive distortions, negative automatic thoughts and dysfunctional attitudes of patients diagnosed with depression. Psychology, Health & Medicine. 2021:1-11

[23] Demir S, Ercan F. The effectiveness of cognitive behavioral therapy-based group counseling on depressive symptomatology, anxiety levels, automatic thoughts, and coping ways Turkish nursing students: A randomized controlled trial. Perspectives in Psychiatric Care. 2022

[24] Kwee CM, Baas JM, van der Flier FE, Groenink L, Duits P, Eikelenboom M, et al. Cannabidiol enhancement of exposure therapy in treatment refractory patients with social anxiety disorder and panic disorder with agoraphobia: A randomised controlled trial. European Neuropsychopharmacology. 2022;**59**:58-67

[25] Riemer H, Noel H. The effect of emotionally-arousing ad appeals on memory: Time and fit matter. International Journal of Advertising. 2021;**40**(7):1024-1046

[26] Jelsma EB, Goosby BJ, Cheadle JE. Do trait psychological characteristics moderate sympathetic arousal to racial discrimination exposure in a natural setting? Psychophysiology. 2021;**58**(4):e13763

[27] Nabi RL, So J, Prestin A, Torres DDP. Media-based emotional coping: Examining the emotional benefits and pitfalls of media consumption. In: Routledge International Handbook of Emotions and Media. Routledge; 2021. pp. 85-101

[28] Smith VM, Watson P, Most SB. Enhanced recognition of emotional images is not affected by post-exposure exercise-induced arousal. Quarterly Journal of Experimental Psychology. 2022;**75**(6):1056-1066

[29] Yao W, Zhang X, Gong Q. The effect of exposure to the natural environment on stress reduction: A meta-analysis. Urban Forestry & Urban Greening. 2021;**57**:126932

[30] Karyotaki E, Efthimiou O, Miguel C, Bermpohl FMG, Furukawa TA,

Cuijpers P, et al. Internet-based cognitive behavioral therapy for depression: A systematic review and individual patient data network meta-analysis. JAMA Psychiatry. 2021;**78**(4):361-371

[31] Sarin F, Wallin L, Widerlöv B. Cognitive behavior therapy for schizophrenia: A meta-analytical review of randomized controlled trials. Nordic Journal of Psychiatry. 2011;**65**(3):162-174

[32] Burns AM, Erickson DH, Brenner CA. Cognitive-behavioral therapy for medication-resistant psychosis: A meta-analytic review. Psychiatric Services. 2014;**65**(7):874-880

[33] Hofmann SG, Asnaani A, Vonk IJ, Sawyer AT, Fang A. The efficacy of cognitive behavioral therapy: A review of meta-analyses. Cognitive Therapy and Research. 2012;**36**(5):427-440

[34] Salkovskis, P. M., Warwick, H. (2001). Meaning, Misinterpretations, and Medicine: A Cognitive-Behavioral Approach to Understanding Health Anxiety and Hypochondriasis.

[35] Van Dijk S, Jeffrey J, Katz MR. A randomized, controlled, pilot study of dialectical behavior therapy skills in a psychoeducational group for individuals with bipolar disorder. Journal of Affective Disorders. 2013;**145**(3):386-393

[36] Afshari B, Dehkordi FJ, Farid AAA, Aramfar B, Balagabri Z, Mohebi M, et al. Study of cognitive behavior therapy versus dialectical behavior therapy on executive function and symptoms reduction in generalized anxiety disorder. Trends in Psychiatry and Psychotherapy. 2022 (ahead of print)

[37] Afshari B, Hasani J. Study of dialectical behavior therapy versus cognitive behavior therapy on emotion regulation and mindfulness in patients with generalized anxiety disorder. Journal of Contemporary Psychotherapy. 2020;**50**(4):305-312

[38] Afshari B, Shiri N, Ghoreishi FS, Valianpour M. Examination and comparison of cognitive and executive functions in clinically stable schizophrenia disorder, bipolar disorder, and major depressive disorder. Depression Research and Treatment. 2020

[39] Rezaie Z, Afshari B, Balagabri Z. Effects of dialectical behavior therapy on emotion regulation, distress tolerance, craving, and depression in patients with opioid dependence disorder. Journal of Contemporary Psychotherapy. 2021:1-10

[40] Linehan MM, Schmidt H, Dimeff LA, Craft JC, Kanter J, Comtois KA. Dialectical behavior therapy for patients with borderline personality disorder and drug-dependence. American Journal on Addictions. 1999;**8**(4):279-292

[41] Linehan MM, Korslund KE, Harned MS, Gallop RJ, Lungu A, Neacsiu AD, et al. Dialectical behavior therapy for high suicide risk in individuals with borderline personality disorder: A randomized clinical trial and component analysis. JAMA Psychiatry. 2015;**72**(5):475-482

[42] Afshari B, Omidi A, Ahmadvand A. Effects of dialectical behavior therapy on executive functions, emotion regulation, and mindfulness in bipolar disorder. Journal of Contemporary Psychotherapy. 2020;**50**(2):123-131

[43] Harley R, Sprich S, Safren S, Jacobo M, Fava M. Adaptation of dialectical behavior therapy skills training group for treatment-resistant depression. The Journal of Nervous and Mental Disease. 2008;**196**(2):136-143

[44] Goldstein TR, Axelson DA, Birmaher B, Brent DA. Dialectical

behavior therapy for adolescents with bipolar disorder: A 1-year open trial. Journal of the American Academy of Child & Adolescent Psychiatry. 2007;**46**(7):820-830

[45] Nelson-Gray RO, Keane SP, Hurst RM, Mitchell JT, Warburton JB, Chok JT, et al. A modified DBT skills training program for oppositional defiant adolescents: Promising preliminary findings. Behaviour Research and Therapy. 2006;**44**(12):1811-1820

[46] Keuthen NJ, Rothbaum BO, Welch SS, Taylor C, Falkenstein M, Heekin M, et al. Pilot trial of dialectical behavior therapy-enhanced habit reversal for trichotillomania. Depression and Anxiety. 2010;**27**(10):953-959

[47] Steil R, Dyer A, Priebe K, Kleindienst N, Bohus M. Dialectical behavior therapy for posttraumatic stress disorder related to childhood sexual abuse: A pilot study of an intensive residential treatment program. Journal of Traumatic Stress. 2011;**24**(1):102-106

[48] Perepletchikova F, Axelrod SR, Kaufman J, Rounsaville BJ, Douglas-Palumberi H, Miller AL. Adapting dialectical behaviour therapy for children: Towards a new research agenda for paediatric suicidal and non-suicidal self-injurious behaviours. Child and Adolescent Mental Health. 2011;**16**(2):116-121

[49] Rajalin M, Wickholm-Pethrus L, Hursti T, Jokinen J. Dialectical behavior therapy-based skills training for family members of suicide attempters. Archives of Suicide Research. 2009;**13**(3):257-263

[50] Evershed S, Tennant A, Boomer D, Rees A, Barkham M, Watson A. Practice-based outcomes of dialectical behaviour therapy (DBT) targeting anger and violence, with male forensic patients: A pragmatic and non-contemporaneous comparison. Criminal Behaviour and Mental Health. 2003;**13**(3):198-213

[51] Sakdalan JA, Shaw J, Collier V. Staying in the here-and-now: A pilot study on the use of dialectical behaviour therapy group skills training for forensic clients with intellectual disability. Journal of Intellectual Disability Research. 2010;**54**(6):568-572

[52] Drossel C, Fisher JE, Mercer V. A DBT skills training group for family caregivers of persons with dementia. Behavior Therapy. 2011;**42**(1):109-119

[53] Segal Z, Williams M, Teasdale J. Mindfulness-based Cognitive Therapy for Depression. Guilford Publications; 2018

[54] Kabat-Zinn J. Mindfulness-based stress reduction (MBSR). Constructivism in the Human Sciences. 2003;**8**(2):73

[55] Kuyken W, Watkins E, Holden E, White K, Taylor RS, Byford S, et al. How does mindfulness-based cognitive therapy work? Behaviour Research and Therapy. 2010;**48**(11):1105-1112

[56] Hayes SC, Hofmann SG. The third wave of cognitive behavioral therapy and the rise of process-based care. World Psychiatry. 2017;**16**(3):245

[57] Grossman P, Niemann L, Schmidt S, Walach H. Mindfulness-based stress reduction and health benefits: A meta-analysis. Journal of Psychosomatic Research. 2004;**57**(1):35-43

[58] Gaboury I, Dobkin P, Roberge P, Beaulieu M-C, Dagenais P, Gervais F, et al. Mindfulness-based reduction stress reduction for patients with rheumatoid arthritis and depressive symptoms: A pilot trial. The International Journal of Whole Person Care. 2020;**7**(1):7-8

[59] Schanche E, Vøllestad J, Binder P-E, Hjeltnes A, Dundas I, Nielsen GH. Participant experiences of change in mindfulness-based stress reduction for anxiety disorders. International Journal of Qualitative Studies on Health and Well-Being. 2020;**15**(1):1776094

[60] Hayes SC, Strosahl KD, Wilson KG. Acceptance and Commitment Therapy. Washington, DC: American Psychological Association; 2009

[61] Hayes SC, Strosahl KD, Wilson KG. Acceptance and Commitment Therapy: The Process and Practice of Mindful Change. Guilford Press; 2011

[62] Hayes SC, Luoma JB, Bond FW, Masuda A, Lillis J. Acceptance and commitment therapy: Model, processes and outcomes. Behaviour Research and Therapy. 2006;**44**(1):1-25

[63] Harris R. ACT Made Simple: An Easy-to-Read Primer on Acceptance and Commitment Therapy. New Harbinger Publications; 2019

[64] Butryn ML, Forman E, Hoffman K, Shaw J, Juarascio A. A pilot study of acceptance and commitment therapy for promotion of physical activity. Journal of Physical Activity & Health. 2011;**8**(4)

[65] Levin M, Hayes SC. Is acceptance and commitment therapy superior to established treatment comparisons. Psychotherapy and Psychosomatics. 2009;**78**(6):380

[66] Wells A, King P. Metacognitive therapy for generalized anxiety disorder: An open trial. Journal of Behavior Therapy and Experimental Psychiatry. 2006;**37**(3):206-212

Chapter 6

The Effect of Physical Activity Intervention on Panic and Anxiety Symptoms in Children, Adolescents and Early Adulthoods: A Meta-Analysis

Lin Wang and Yihao Liu

Abstract

Physical activity is believed to promote mental health. However, research has not yet reached a consensus on whether physical activity declines panic and anxiety symptoms in children, adolescents, and early adulthoods. The current chapter carried out a meta-analysis to investigate the association between physical activity and panic/anxiety based on the Preferred Reporting Items for Systematic Reviews and Meta-Analyses (PRISMA) 2020 guidelines. Search is conducted on 22nd April 2022, which follow databases: MEDLINE (Ovid), EMBASE, Web of Science, Cochrane Central Register of Controlled Trials, and SPORTDiscus. Fifteen articles ($N = 994$) were identified and included, where four studies reported measurement in panic symptoms and fourteen studies reported measurement in anxiety symptoms. The meta-analysis among the pooled effect sizes demonstrated a small significant effect of physical activity intervention reducing panic disorder ($d = -.45$, $SE = .12$, $Z = -3.65$, $p < .001$) and a middle effect reducing anxiety ($d = -.51$, $SE = .15$, $Z = -3.38$, $p < .001$) in children, adolescents and early adulthoods. Age or gender ratio was not found to be significant in predicting the effect sizes. More evidence is required to produce a solid conclusion.

Keywords: panic disorder, anxiety disorder, physical activity intervention, children and adolescents, systematic review

1. Introduction

Physical activity (PA) is one of the most accessible interventions for anxiety disorders for the public, whereas few systematic research has been done to examine its efficacy. PA is defined as a movement that causes an increase in energy expenditure in the movement of people [1], including walking, running, doing housework, jogging, or other sports that are defined as PA behaviour [2, 3]. Dollman et al. (2015) have classified PA intensity with metabolic equivalent (MET) as light PA (MET: 0–2.99), moderate-to-vigorous PA (MET:3–5.99), and vigorous PA (MET: ≥6) through a scale of energy expenditure [4–6]. PA intervention aims to promote the health of people through exercise training, sports and habit of PA [7, 8]. A PA intervention study should specify the processing target (e.g., children, adolescents, or some clinic population), PA type (e.g., aerobic exercise, resistance exercise, or yoga), PA intensity (e.g., light, moderator, moderator-to-vigorous), PA frequency (e.g., three sessions per week, 60 minutes per session), PA duration (e.g., three months, 1 years), and outcome measurement [9]. The PA intervention research is easier to quantify and more accessible to the generalised population. It is also found to benefit mental health. Therefore, research is also focused on the effect of PA intervention on panic disorder.

For example, Ensari, Petruzzello [10] conducted an RCT experiment to deliver a 40-minute yoga programme for eighteen participants with high-anxious. The result suggested a significant main effect of the task on panic and respiratory measures ($p < .05$). When collapsed over inhibition task and condition, there was a small reduction in cognitive anxiety from baseline to immediately post and 1-h post-condition ($p < .05$) [10]. Similarly, Naderi, Naderi [11] investigated the effect of physical exercise on anxiety among victims of child abuse and reported a significant reduction in anxiety ($p < .001$). Accordingly, the author argued that such improvement is comparable to empirically supported treatments for panic and GAD. However, such effects of PA intervention on panic disorder used a variety of PA types, intensity levels, or frequency and, therefore, produced isolated effects. The effect of PA could vary regarding individual differences, such as age and gender [12]. A most recent systematic review in 2022 tended to examine the effect of regular exercise interventions on the panic disorder in adults. They only retrieved eight studies in this field and demonstrated no clear evidence suggesting whether regular exercise programs (at least two 20-minute sessions per week for at least six weeks) reduce panic-related symptoms. The study argued for more RCT studies to support more robust and clear evidence for better understanding [11].

Moreover, there were even fewer studies focused on the effect of PA intervention on the panic disorder or general anxiety disorder (GAD) in children and adolescents, respectively. This may be because it is difficult to categorise different anxiety disorders among children. Furthermore, there is a lack of tools to measure child panic in laboratory settings. For example, there is the anxiety scale for children with autism spectrum disorder, revised children's manifest anxiety scale and social anxiety scale for children to measure anxiety disorder in children and adolescents [9, 13, 14], whereas the panic disorder is measured based on the sensitivity of anxiety scales in children and adolescents [15]. These unclear concepts may increase the research difficulty, which supports the evidence for PA intervention on panic disorder in children and adolescents. Therefore, this chapter aims to carry out a quantitative review to clarify and explore the evidence in this area. Moreover, the secondary objective is to investigate the effect of PA intervention on anxiety disorder in children and adolescents.

The previous Machado, Telles [11] review obtained a similar outcome measurement to examine the effect of PA on anxiety disorder. Their target sample did not limit the population age, which means there is no evidence that physical activities affect panic and anxiety disorder in children and adolescents. Consequently, the current analysis aims 1) to summarise and explain the potential impact of PA interventions on panic symptoms and critically comment on the research that exists and 2) to analyse the effect of PA intervention on panic and anxiety symptoms in children, adolescents and early adulthood, through meta-analysis, which provides reference evidence for further research.

2. Method

2.1 Materials and methods protocol and registration

The study is based on the Preferred Reporting Items for Systematic Reviews and Meta-Analyses (PRISMA) 2020 guidelines. A protocol for this review was registered with PROSPERO (CRD42022334054).

2.2 Search strategy and databases

Search is conducted on 22nd April 2022, which follow databases: MEDLINE (Ovid), EMBASE, Web of Science, Cochrane Central Register of Controlled Trials, and SPORTDiscus. Search terms based on the PICO format (participants/population, intervention/exposure, comparison, outcome) were divided, and adjusted according to the respective databases' Thesaurus and Medical Subject Headings (MeSH) terms (Bramer et al., 2018) through Ovid. Articles must be available in English, there will be no restriction on the publication period. The full list of search terms is provided in Supplementary Material 1.

2.3 Eligibility criteria

The inclusion criteria of the current analysis were: 1) Population: studies included participants who primarily exhibited panic or anxiety symptoms or were diagnosed with panic or anxiety disorders in children, adolescents (5–19 years) and early adulthoods (19–22 years). Participants may present secondary comorbid other illnesses, such as diabetes; 2) Intervention: studies applied regular PA intervention (i.e. walk, jog, aerobic, strength, or multimodal training), which is prescribed to reduce panic disorder or GAD, social anxiety disorder, obsessive–compulsive disorder, post-traumatic stress disorder, and agoraphobia. PA interventions can be combined with other treatment procedures were also included; 3) Comparators: studies included a control group as a comparator, which is not received the PA intervention delivery; 4) Outcomes: studies that took panic symptoms or panic disorder as the primary outcome. And the second outcome was anxiety symptoms, GAD, social anxiety disorder, obsessive–compulsive disorder, post-traumatic stress disorder, or agoraphobia; 5) Study Design: studies carried out in randomised trials (RCT) comparing an intervention(s) encompassing PA with a group(s) without PA intervention or encompassing PA at the baseline with post PA intervention.

The exclusion criteria were: 1) studies reported in non-English language; 2) studies reported insufficient information to estimate effect size or other essential data.

2.4 Article selection and data extraction

Study selection: Data will be formatted in RIS format and will be managed using the endnote software. PRISMA 2020 guidelines will be applied for reporting the screening process [16]. Two researchers will undertake the removal process through an independent screen. Firstly, all duplicate articles will be removed before reviewing titles and abstracts. Those not fitting the inclusion criteria will be removed. Then, full-text versions will be collected when the articles meet the screening criteria. Discussions with a third reviewer will resolve discrepancies between the two independent reviewers.

Data extraction: Two independent reviewers will extract the following four data dimensions. Including fundamental characteristics (e.g., author, public year, country, population, sample, age, sex, weight status), intervention characteristics (e.g., PA intensity/frequency/duration, intervention program), methodology (e.g., data analysis method), and effect size.

2.5 Risk-of-bias (quality) assessment

Two reviewers will independently score the studies according to the National Institutes of Health study quality assessment tool for Quality Assessment of Controlled Intervention Studies from the National Heart, Lung, and Blood Institute (https://www.nhlbi.nih.gov/health-topics/study-quality-assessment-tools). The quality assessment focused on the specification of eligibility criteria, generalisability, intervention description, outcome assessment and incomplete data [17]. There were 14 items assessed in the quality assessment, as shown in Appendix S1. The tool does not assign numeric values or definite judgements of the quality of the studies, although it has good, fair, and poor results. Good quality studies have less bias risk and are more valid. A fair study is prone to some bias but insufficient to invalidate its findings. A poor study has a high-risk of bias and is considered invalid [18]. The results of quality assessment are presented in **Table 1**.

2.6 Effect size estimation

The studies we aimed to include in the current analysis were RCTs with both between-subject, within-subject and mixed designs. Consequently, a combined effect size of standard mean difference (Cohen's d) was calculated for each study to produce a pooled effect size based on the improved method provided in Morris [19]. Firstly, the effect size of studies reported only median and interquartile range was estimated based on the improved formula [20, 21], where d refers to Cohen's d; q1 refers to the first quartile; q3 refers to the third quartile:

$$d = \frac{q_3 - q_1}{1.35}$$

Moreover, studies reported pre-calculated Cohen's d without providing the mean or standard deviation was estimated standard error using the 95% confidence interval for meta-analysis weighting [22], where SE refers to standard error, CL_{up} and CL_{low} refer to the upper and the lower bound of the confidence interval, respectively:

$$SE = \frac{CL_{up} - CL_{low}}{3.92}$$

The effect sizes were from between-subject design, within-subject design and mixed design studies were extracted, converted and matched to Cohen's d with an online converter tool 'Psychometrica' (https://www.psychometrica.de/effect_size.html), which follows the method proposed in Morris [19] and Lakens [23].

2.7 Statistical data analysis

The statistical analysis was carried out in STATA v.17. The estimated effect sizes of adolescent panic and anxiety were pooled in a quantitative meta-analysis in a random

Study	1	2	3	4	5	6	7	8	9	10	11	12	13	14	overall
Kenis-Coskun et al., 2022	Y	Y	Y	NR	NR	Y	Y	Y	Y	Y	Y	Y	Y	Y	Good
Tanksale et al., 2021	Y	Y	N	N	N	Y	Y	Y	N	Y	Y	NR	NA	Y	Fair
Nazari et al., 2020	Y	Y	N	N	N	Y	Y	Y	NR	Y	Y	Y	Y	Y	Fair
Romero-Pérez et al., 2020	Y	Y	N	N	N	Y	Y	Y	Y	Y	Y	NR	Y	Y	Fair
Yu et al., 2020	Y	Y	N	N	N	N	Y	Y	Y	Y	Y	Y	Y	Y	Fair
Mucke et al., 2020	Y	Y	N	N	N	Y	Y	Y	Y	Y	Y	Y	NA	Y	Good
Akko et al., 2020	Y	Y	N	N	N	Y	Y	Y	Y	Y	Y	Y	Y	Y	Good
Luna et al., 2019	Y	Y	N	N	N	Y	Y	Y	Y	Y	Y	NR	Y	Y	Fair
Naderi et al., 2019	Y	Y	N	N	N	Y	Y	Y	Y	Y	Y	NR	Y	Y	Fair
Ensari et al., 2019	Y	N	N	NR	NR	Y	Y	Y	Y	Y	Y	NR	Y	Y	Fair
Polis et al., 2017	Y	Y	N	N	N	Y	Y	Y	NR	Y	Y	NR	NA	Y	Fair
Smits et al., 2009	Y	N	NR	NR	NR	Y	Y	Y	Y	Y	Y	NR	Y	Y	Fair
Broman-Fulks & Storey, 2008	Y	N	NR	NR	NR	Y	Y	Y	Y	Y	Y	NR	Y	Y	Fair
Lindwall et al., 2005	Y	Y	N	N	N	Y	N	N	N	NA	Y	NR	Y	Y	Poor
Crew et al., 2004	Y	Y	N	N	N	Y	Y	Y	Y	N	Y	NR	NA	Y	Fair

Table 1.
Summary of quality of included studies.

effect model and Cohen's d to determine the overall effect among the studies. A significant result of this analysis indicates that there was a significant effect of physical activities/exercise on adolescent panic or anxiety across the studies. The effect size is considered small when SMD is between 0.2 and 0.5, medium when it is between 0.5 and 0.8, and large when it is above 0.8 [24].

Then, a heterogeneity test of the available data was carried out with the random effect model. A non-significant result in the heterogeneity test would mean that the effect sizes were homogenous and measured a consistent effect on the same side. The heterogeneity I^2 is considered moderate when $I^2 > 50\%$, and it is considered high when $I^2 > 75\%$ [21]. Egger's regression-based tests were then used to assess the publication bias. A significant result in this test would suggest potential publication bias in the current analysis.

Finally, exploratory meta-regression analyses were performed on the available characteristic data, including age, gender and intervention duration, to determine potential predictors of the current effect. The research method would be entered into subgroup analysis to determine whether the study design made a difference in the overall effect.

3. Results

3.1 Data acquisition

As shown in Appendix 2, keywords searching in MEDLINE (Ovid), EMBASE, Web of Science, Cochrane Central Register of Controlled Trials, and SportDiscus resulted in 1691 articles. After reviewing, based on inclusion criteria, twelve studies were identified, and four studies were excluded based on exclusion criteria, leaving eight studies for the meta-analysis. The included 11 studies were all RCTs in different designs (within-subject, between-subject and mixed design).

3.2 Characteristics of included literature

As shown in **Table 2**, 15 RCT studies with sufficient data were included. Among these studies, 14 obtained anxiety measurements, including social anxiety disorder [14, 25, 26] and GAD [10, 13, 27–32], and 4 studies obtained panic measurements [10, 31–33]. There were 994 participants included in total, and 478 and 354 participants were allocated in the intervention and control groups, respectively. The mean age of the participants was 13.21 ± 4.16 years old, ranging from 8 to 24 years old. Physical activity intervention duration was from a minimum of 2 weeks to 8 months, and frequency was 2 or 3 sessions per week, with two studies performing a one-session intervention [10, 34]. Two studies also provided discussion and reflection sessions after the physical activity sessions [34, 35] and two studies were conducted on the school campus [14, 28].

IG = intervention group; CG = control group; Pre-I: pre-intervention; Post-I: post-intervention; s/w = sessions per week; NR = not reported; NA = not applicable; ASC-ASD: Anxiety Scale for Children–Autism Spectrum Disorder RCMAS = Revised Children's Manifest Anxiety Scale; SAQ-C24 = Social Anxiety Scale for Children; SAS-A = Social Anxiety Scale for Adolescents; STAI = State–Trait Anxiety Inventory; SAI = State Anxiety Inventory; SPAS = Social Physique Anxiety Scale; RCADS = Anxiety and Depression Scale in Children-Revised; API = Acute Panic Inventory; ASI-R = Anxiety Sensitivity Index-Revised. The sports type are labelled in bold.

Study	Overall sample	IG sample Pre-I (Post-I)	CG sample Pre-I (Post-I)	Overall age (SD)	Female sample	IG content	CG content	Frequency (Duration)	Panic and anxiety measurement	Study Design	Intensity measurement
Kenis-Coskun et al., 2022	28	14 (14)	14 (14)	9.90 (1.91)	20	Multiple rehabilitation exercises repeated 10 times each: Corner Pectoral Stretch; Scapular Retraction with External Rotation; Triceps Brachii Strengthening; Biceps Strengthening Exercise; Biceps Strengthening Exercise; Lateral Abdominal Muscle Strengthening Exercise; Push Up; Back Extensors Strengthening.	NR	3 s/w (12 weeks)	RCADS	Mixed	NA
Tanksale et al., 2021	61	31 (31)	30 (30)	9.44 (1.35)	22	The lead researcher delivered the Yoga program face-to-face to all participants on the university campus within a group of less than 5 parent–child dyads.	Participants were randomly allocated to a waiting list without receiving intervention	1 s/w (6 weeks)	ASC-ASD	Between-subject	NA
Nazari et al., 2020	40	20 (20)	20 (20)	11.11 (2.29)	NR	20 mins of Pilates exercises & 20 mins of body weight-bearing exercise & 20 mins aerobic exercises (V-forward, V-back & march)	NR	3 s/w (16 weeks)	RCMAS	Mixed	Heart rate

Study	Overall sample	IG sample Pre-I (Post-I)	CG sample Pre-I (Post-I)	Overall age (SD)	Female sample	IG content	CG content	Frequency (Duration)	Panic and anxiety measurement	Study Design	Intensity measurement
Romero-Pérez et al., 2020	105	54 (54)	51 (51)	9.88 (0.83)	60	5-min warm-up, a 40-min aerobic exercise	The CG participants continued with their usual activities at the end of the classes	2 s/w (20 weeks)	RCMAS	Mixed	NA
Yu et al., 2020	188	106 (99)	82 (72)	9.8 (0.7)	35	20-min class recess in the morning and one extra gym class (40 min) after school in the afternoon, including Jogging 20 min in the morning break every weekday; Rope skipping 40 min on Monday and Thursday; Playing badminton 40 min on Wednesday and Friday; 200-m relay race 40 min on Tuesday.	Children in the control school followed their usual practice with no extra intervention	(weekday daily) 5 s/w (8 months)	SAQ-C24	Mixed	NA
Mucke et al., 2020	60	30 (NA)	30 (NA)	17.9 (1.24)	0	The exercise group performed an exercise session at moderate intensity on a bicycle ergometer (30 mins)	During the next 30 mins, the control group read an article from a magazine of their choice	One session	STAI	Between-subject	Heart Rate

Study	Overall sample	IG sample Pre-I (Post-I)	CG sample Pre-I (Post-I)	Overall age (SD)	Female sample	IG content	CG content	Frequency (Duration)	Panic and anxiety measurement	Study Design	Intensity measurement
Akko et al., 2020	44	23 (23)	21 (21)	9.35 (0.6)	39	45 min after school running and running-based games of moderate-intensity	preadolescent children participated in assisted homework sessions to prevent attention bias and to control for retest effects	3 s/w (10 weeks)	STAI	Mixed	NA
Luna et al., 2019	113	69 (69)	44 (44)	13.82 (0.79)	49	55-minute sessions volleyball sessions, including warming-up, training and friendly matches and regular stage competition; Meetings for comprehension and reflection with the intervention of the responsibility roles	Traditional collective sport (basketball) with a conventional teaching style in which the teachers directed all tasks without students' participation	2–3 s/w (6 weeks)	SAS-A	Mixed	NA
Naderi et al., 2019	22	11 (11)	11 (11)	8 to 11	22	Aerobic dancing: Warming up (10–15 min); Basic movements (35–40 min); Cooling down (10 min)	Not receiving any intervention	3 s/w(8 weeks)	STAI	Mixed	NA

Study	Overall sample	IG sample Pre-I (Post-I)	CG sample Pre-I (Post-I)	Overall age (SD)	Female sample	IG content	CG content	Frequency (Duration)	Panic and anxiety measurement	Study Design	Intensity measurement
Ensari et al., 2019	18	9 (9)	9 (9)	22.1 (5.0)	18	40 min Yoga session, which was designed based on published recommendations under the guidance of an instructor with the specific order of poses	Stretching exercises	One session	API & SAI	Mixed	Heart Rate
Polis et al., 2017	23	12 (5)	11 (8)	11 to 18	NR	Evening yoga session led by yoga instructor	NR	2 s/w (6 weeks)	STAI	Mixed	NA
Smits et al., 2009	92	48 (48)	44 (44)	19.43 (1.31)	51	20 min treadmill exercise on a computer-controlled treadmill, maintaining 70% of max heart rate	20-min resting period	One session	API	Mixed	Heart Rate
Broman-Fulks & Storey, 2008	24	12 (12)	12 (12)	19.04 (1.90)	19	20 min aerobic exercise: treadmill running	Report to the lab at the same time but no exercise	3 s/w (2 weeks)	ASI-R	Mixed	Heart Rate
Lindwall et al., 2005	110	56 (27)	54 (35)	16.35 (1.56)	110	Preferred multiple aerobics exercises (45 min) and discussion (15 min), including water aerobics, step-up, badminton, kickboxing, spinning dancing, climbing, bowling, karate, jujitsu, yoga and different ballgames	Control group were put on a waiting list with no forms of alternative activities organised	2 s/w (24 weeks)	SPAS	Mixed	NA

Study	Overall sample	IG sample Pre-I (Post-I)	CG sample Pre-I (Post-I)	Overall age (SD)	Female sample	IG content	CG content	Frequency (Duration)	Panic and anxiety measurement	Study Design	Intensity measurement
Crew et al., 2004	66	66 (66)	NA	NR (Grade 4)	33	The aerobic group exercised by means of stationary cycling, track running, and jumping on a minitrampoline. The physical activity group engaged in a variety of physical activities such as shooting baskets for skill improvement, playing a common children's game called foursquare, and walking	NA	3 s/w (6 weeks)	STAI	Within-subject	Heart Rate
Overall	994	561 (488)	433 (371)	13.21 (4.16)	478 (51.3%)						

Table 2.
Characteristics of included studies.

NA: not applicable, NR: not reported, CD: cannot determine, overall of Good: more than 10Y (NA = Y), Fair 8 to 10Y, Poor: Below 8.

3.3 Risk-of-bias (quality) assessment

Overall, three reports showed good quality, whereas most studies were fair. We can find that in terms of random methods, most of the studies do not report the process of random sampling and there are basically no studies that apply computer random sampling methods. In addition, the information reported on the sample power is relatively lacking.

3.4 Effect of PA intervention on panic

Main effect. As shown in **Figure 1**, the pooled effect size revealed a significant overall effect of physical activity on panic symptoms from four studies (Random effects; $d = -.45$, SE = .12, Z = −3.65, $p < .001$). Estimation of the homogeneity suggested that the chance of inconsistent distribution of the effect sizes was not significant, Q(3) = 1.36, $p = .715$. Sensitivity analysis revealed small-to-no heterogeneity across the effect sizes of the studies, $I^2 = 0.00\%$. These results mean that the effect sizes across four studies suggested a significant small effect of physical activity in reducing panic symptoms among children, adolescents and early adulthood compared to the controls.

Publication bias. As shown in **Figure 2**, Egger's regression-based tests suggested no estimated publication bias, $\beta = .57$, SE = .1,06 t = .54, $p = .644$. One study with small sample size (N = 24) reported high standard error [32].

Exploratory meta-regression. Age and gender ratios were entered into meta-regression analysis to determine potential predictors for the combined effect sizes. As summarised in **Table 3**, meta-regression analysis suggested no significant predictor for the combined effect sizes of current studies, $R^2 = .00$, Qw(2) = 1.35, $p = .508$. This means that age or gender ratios were not significant predictors of the current pooled effect sizes.

3.5 Effect of PA intervention on anxiety

Main effect. As shown in **Figure 3**, the pooled effect size revealed a significant overall effect of physical activity on anxiety from 14 studies (Random effects;

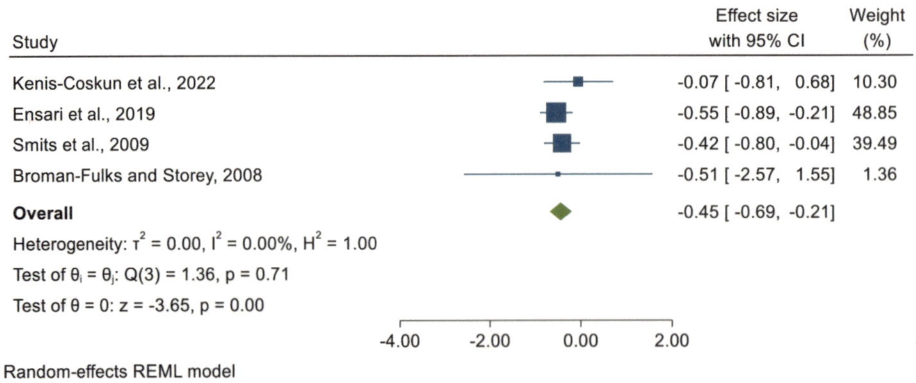

Figure 1.
The forest plot of the effect size of physical activity on panic in children, adolescents and early adulthood.

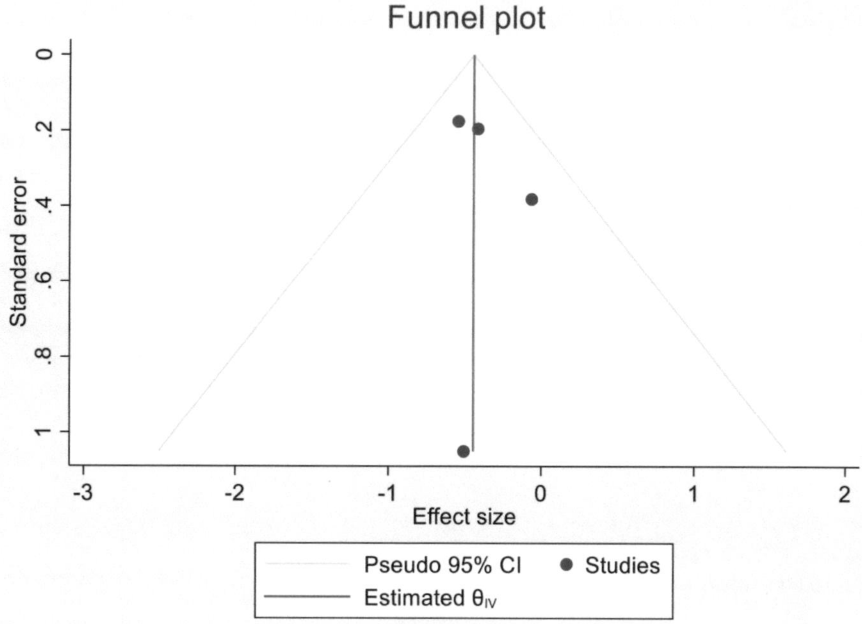

Figure 2.
Funnel plot of the effect size estimates of physical activity on the panic symptoms in children and adolescents.

Predictor	Coefficient B	SE	95% CI	z	*p*
Age	−.03	.03	[−.11 .04]	−.99	.325
Gender Ratio (Female)	−.06	.66	[−1.35 1.23]	0.09	.927

Table 3.
Meta-regression analysis on age and gender predicting pooled effect sizes of PA intervention reducing panic disorder.

$d = -.51$, SE = .15, Z = −3.38, $p < .001$). Estimation of the homogeneity suggested that the chance of inconsistent distribution of the effect sizes was not significant, Q(13) = 20.83, $p = .076$. Sensitivity analysis revealed moderate-to-small heterogeneity across the effect sizes of the studies, $I^2 = 47.52\%$. These results mean that the effect sizes across 14 studies suggested a significant medium effect of physical activity in reducing anxiety among children and adolescents compared to the controls.

Publication bias. As shown in **Figure 4**, Egger's regression-based tests suggested no estimated publication bias, $\beta = -.58$, SE = .63, t = −.92, $p = .377$. One study was outside of the funnel [10], of which the recorded main effect was a three-way interaction (pre vs. post & PA vs. Control & inhalation task 1 vs. task 2 vs. task 3). Such a small sample size (N = 18) and physiological measurement design (inhalation task) reported a greater effect size and small standard error comparing to other self-report questionnaires. It only counted 8.34% of the weight, which was not considered producing bias to the overall result. And another study reported high standard error because the sample size was very small (N = 23) [30].

Exploratory meta-regression and subgroup analysis. Age and gender ratios were entered into meta-regression analysis to determine potential predictors for the

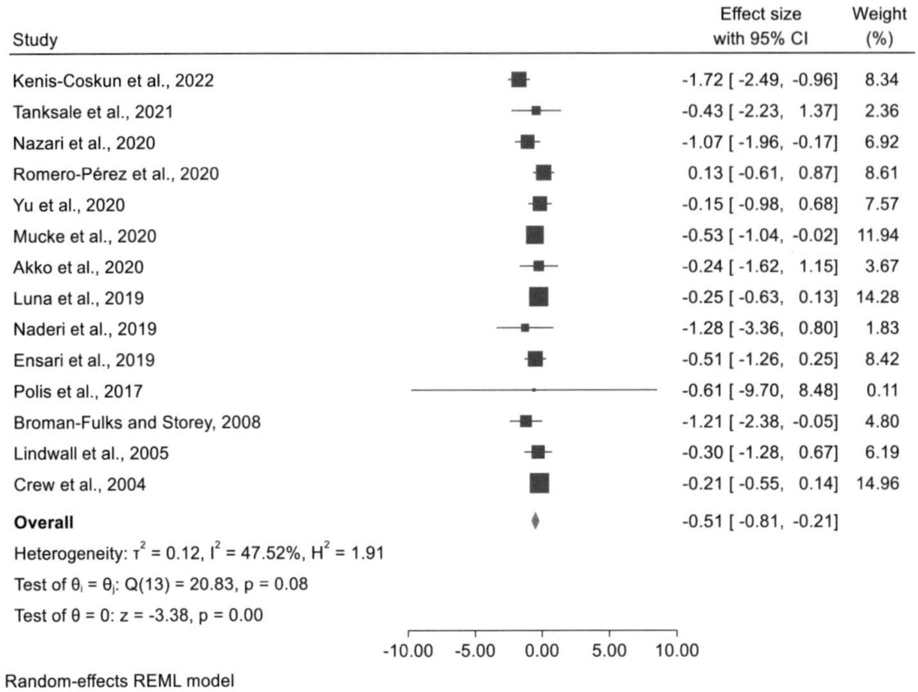

Figure 3.
The forest plot of the effect size of physical activity on anxiety disorder in children and adolescents.

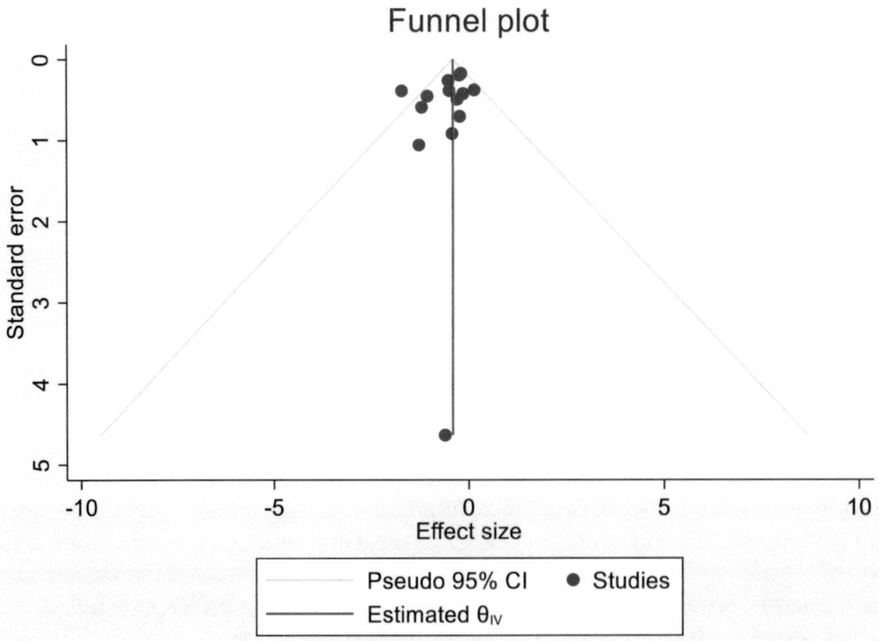

Figure 4.
Funnel plot of the effect size estimates of physical activity on anxiety disorder in children and adolescents.

combined effect sizes. Meta-regression analysis suggested no significant predictor for the combined effect sizes of current studies, $R^2 = .00$, $Qw(2) = .29$, $p = .865$. This means that age or gender ratios were not significant predictors of the current pooled effect sizes.

The research method (mixed-design vs. between-subject & within-subject design) was entered into subgroup analysis to determine whether the main effect changed between the two interactive groups. No significant group difference in homogeneity was identified in either research method, $Qb(1) = 1.26$, $p = .26$.

4. Discussion

The current chapter carried out a meta-analysis on 15 reports to investigate the pooled effect sizes of PA intervention on panic and anxiety symptoms among children, adolescents and early adulthood. Compared to the controls, we reported a small effect of PA on reducing panic symptoms and a middle effect on reducing anxiety symptoms. To our knowledge, this is the first study to summarise the effect of PA on panic and anxiety symptoms in children, adolescents and early adulthood with meta-analysis.

The primary finding of the current meta-analysis is that the pooled effect sizes from 4 reports yielded a significant small effect ($d = -.45$) of PA intervention in reducing panic symptoms. This means PA obtains such potential to be used in therapeutic intervention for panic in children, adolescents and early adulthoods. The mechanism of PA affecting panic symptoms was suggested to be related to the metabolism of CO_2 and lactate. Accordingly, CO_2 and lactate hydrolysed into HCO3- were found to moderate the blood pH level and influence brain acidosis [35]. Specifically, such change in pH level and brain acidosis is related to the activation of the amygdala and, furthermore, regulates the reaction of fear [36, 37]. Here, we would not discuss the biochemical pathology further but highlight the importance of CO_2 and lactate. Empirical evidence suggested that patients with panic disorder were found to have chronically low end-tidal CO_2 [38] and, vice versa, CO_2 inhalation reduces panic symptoms [39]. Similarly, early literature reported an increased lactate level among panic patients [40, 41]. As a result, regulating the brain acidosis condition is believed to attenuate panic symptoms. Apart from direct CO_2 inhalation, appropriate physical activity also regulates CO_2 inhalation and lactate levels, eventually balancing the blood pH and brain acidosis, which is potentially the mechanism of how PA intervention works.

However, it is very important to bear in mind that this result is very primal and exploratory because it was summarised from four reports with limited sample sizes, of which one study targeted children (N = 28) [33], two studies targeted adolescents (N = 92; N = 24, respectively) [31, 32] and one study targeted early adulthoods (N = 18; age mean = 22.1) [10]. There is, to date, indeed a shortage of evidence in this field. A most recent 2022 systematic review only identified eight studies testing PA intervention's effect on panic disorder among adults [11] and argued for more evidence. On the one hand, it is difficult to recruit children with panic symptoms or diagnosed with panic disorder and deliver interventions for them. Unlike general anxiety symptoms, panic disorder is often clinically diagnosed and needs to be treated with extra caution. On the other hand, the tool to measure panic symptoms are limited among children. The experiments included in the current analysis used measurements, including API, RCAD and ASI-R [10, 31–33]. Among these scales, RCAD and

ASI-R are developed for anxiety and only address panic symptoms in their subscales, which were not specifically developed for panic disorder. API was developed for panic symptoms but not aimed at children. It is important to evaluate the assessment tool because the panic among children and adolescents could differ between ages [42]. In comparison, another scale developed after 2014 to measure panic symptoms, namely the Panic Disorder Severity Scale for Children, adapted for adolescents from 11 to 17 years old [43], and used in some studies testing the effect of CBT on panic disorder. Future studies could consider testing the effect of PA on children's panic with suitable assessments.

The secondary finding of the current analysis is that PA intervention had a middle effect ($d = -.51$) in reducing anxiety among children and adolescents. The mechanism of PA reducing anxiety symptoms could be similar to panic symptoms, as mentioned earlier. However, it is noticeable that only four isolated effects were found significant among the included reports in which Kenis-Coskun, Aksoy [33] applied repeated rehabilitation exercises, Nazari, Shabani [13] applied continuous aerobic & resistance exercise intervention, Mücke, Ludyga [34] applied only one session of aerobic exercise at moderate intensity on the bicycle ergometer., and Ensari, Petruzzello [10] applied one Yoga session. A possible reason is that most of these experiments were conducted using a mixed design, with comparisons between experiment and control groups and within the experiment groups. Studies may have reported isolated pronounced effects between the experiment and control group or within the experiment groups, whereas the interaction was not significant [28] or not reported [9, 13, 25, 26, 29, 30]. Only one study reported no effect at all [27]. The data extracted from these studies reflected more combined effects than isolated between-group or within-group effects [19]. Subgroup analysis was also carried out to determine the potential difference between mixed-design and non-mixed design studies (only between-subject or within-subject designs), and no difference was identified between the effect sizes. Consequently, this result should be considered to reflect the actual effects of PA intervention on reducing anxiety.

Knowing that PA intervention reduces panic and anxiety symptoms across the empirical evidence, the next question is what type of exercise produces an optimal effect. The current meta-analysis could not perform the proper subgroup analysis to determine the best PA type due to insufficient data inclusion. Among the 15 studies, three studies applied resistance training, including push up [33], weight-lifting [13] and treadmill exercises [31], whereas others applied aerobic exercise in groups or individually. Among which, the push up and weight-lifting seems to produced the large and significant effect sizes reducing anxiety symptoms ($d = -1.72$, $p < .001$; $d = -1.07$, $p = .002$, respectively) [13, 33]. The effect of resistance training seemed somewhat contradictive to the mechanism in which the high lactate level could induce panic and anxiety symptoms when such anaerobic exercise produces lactate. There are two possible reasons to explain this. One possible reason is that only lactate in the brain induces the change in brain acidosis that leads to panic and anxiety symptoms [44], whereas muscle lactate produced by anaerobic exercise is independent of that in the brain [45]. It is the blood lactate which influences brain acidosis. The second reason is that the participants were measured almost immediately after the PA intervention cooled down, where the blood lactate level remained still. Hiscock, Dawson [46] tested 4 different types of weight-lifting technic to investigate the difference in muscle activation and blood lactate. The blood lactate was measured immediately after the exercise and no change in blood lactate was detected with a significant difference in muscle activation. Consequently, blood lactate was not influenced by different exercise intensities if measured immdiately after the intervention. Hypothetically, it is the regulation of CO_2 during PA that potentially attenuates panic and anxiety symptoms. Future studies could compare, first, the effect of breathing practice from CBT and PA intervention with controlled blood lactate levels. Second, future studies could investigate the long-term effect of resistance training on blood lactate and panic & anxiety symptoms.

The last point to make is that the current meta-regression analysis did not suggest evidence of whether individual differences predicted the pooled effect sizes. Although it was argued in other literature that gender or age could moderate the effect of PA [12]. Previous literature reported gender differences in PA index as age grows [47], and more mature adolescents have more autonomy in PA than children [48], such that they can initiate behaviours that enhance the positive effects of PA on anxiety. As a result, the benefits of PA on depression and anxiety may increase with age. However, the current meta-regression analysis failed to demonstrate such effects on gender or age. One possible reason is that there were only 15 experiments identified in this study, which obtained limited power to detect any individual difference. Thirteen studies reported their gender ratio, and 12 reported the distribution of age. More studies are required to investigate individual differences' role in the effect of PA intervention on anxiety and panic symptoms.

This meta-analysis has several limitations. Firstly, we used Cohen's d rather than Hedges' g to estimate the SMD, which the results might be biased in small sample studies. The reason to pick Cohen's d was that some studies already reported pre-calculated Cohen's d and did not provide sufficient information (N, mean, SD) to carry out transformation or bias correction. With limited numbers of the study identified, it would be impossible to exclude them from the analysis, and this could only be solved by including more studies with sufficient data. Secondly, the current study did not control the comorbidity among children and adolescents, which could affect the outcome of physical activities on panic and anxiety symptoms. As a result, the current results were very primal and exploratory, which should be considered cautiously.

Conclusions

The current meta-analysis reported a small effect of PA intervention on reducing panic symptoms and a middle effect on reducing anxiety symptoms in children, adolescents and early adulthood. Meta-regression analysis did not support age or gender predictors of the pooled effect size. More studies in this field are required to produce a more solid conclusion.

Acknowledgements

We thank all of the staff who contributed their time to our research.

Funding

China Scholarship Council and University of Exeter PhD Scholarship.

Appendices and nomenclature

Appendix 1 Search strategy of systematic review.
Appendix 2 Flow chart of studies retrieved and screened according to the PRISMA.
Appendix 3 Characteristics of included studies.docx.
Appendix 4 Summary of quality of included studies.
Appendix 5 Meta-analysis of raw data.

Author details

Lin Wang[1,2*†] and Yihao Liu[3†]

1 Sports Department, Guilin University of Electronic Technology, China

2 Sport and Health Science Department, University of Exeter, UK

3 Psychology Department, University of Exeter, UK

*Address all correspondence to: lw679@exeter.ac.uk

† Both authors contributed equally to the chapter.

References

[1] Caspersen CJ, Powell KE, Christenson GM. Physical activity, exercise, and physical fitness: Definitions and distinctions for health-related research. Public Health Reports. 1985;**100**(2):126

[2] Kandola AA et al. Impact of replacing sedentary behaviour with other movement behaviours on depression and anxiety symptoms: A prospective cohort study in the UK biobank. BMC Medicine. 2021;**19**(1):133

[3] Cescon M et al. Activity detection and classification from wristband accelerometer data collected on people with type 1 diabetes in free-living conditions. Computers in Biology and Medicine. 2021;**135**:104633

[4] Hills AP, Mokhtar N, Byrne NM. Assessment of physical activity and energy expenditure: An overview of objective measures. Frontiers in Nutrition. 2014;**1**:5

[5] Trost SG et al. Comparison of accelerometer cut points for predicting activity intensity in youth. Medicine and Science in Sports and Exercise. 2011;**43**(7):1360-1368

[6] Howe CA et al. Comparison of accelerometer-based cut-points for Children's physical activity: Counts vs steps. Children (Basel). 2018;**5**(8):105

[7] Bess HM et al. Efficacy of an individualized, motivationally-tailored physical activity intervention. The Society of Behavioral Medicine. 1998;**20**(3):174-180

[8] Cavallo DN et al. A social media-based physical activity intervention: A randomized controlled trial. American Journal of Preventive Medicine. 2012;**43**(5):527-532

[9] Tanksale R et al. Evaluating the effects of a yoga-based program integrated with third-wave cognitive behavioral therapy components on self-regulation in children on the autism spectrum: A pilot randomized controlled trial. Autism. 2021;**25**(4):995-1008

[10] Ensari I, Petruzzello SJ, Motl RW. The effects of acute yoga on anxiety symptoms in response to a carbon dioxide inhalation task in women. Complementary Therapies in Medicine. 2019;**47**:102230

[11] Machado S et al. Can regular physical exercise be a treatment for panic disorder? A systematic review. Expert Review of Neurotherapeutics. 2022;**22**(1):53-64

[12] Bhui K, Fletcher A. Common mood and anxiety states: Gender differences in the protective effect of physical activity. Social Psychiatry and Psychiatric Epidemiology. 2000;**35**(1):28-35

[13] Nazari M, Shabani R, Dalili S. The effect of concurrent resistance-aerobic training on serum cortisol level, anxiety, and quality of life in pediatric type 1 diabetes. Journal of pediatric endocrinology & metabolism : JPEM. 2020;**33**(5):599-604

[14] Yu HJ et al. Improving the metabolic and mental health of children with obesity: A school-based nutrition education and physical activity intervention in Wuhan, China. Nutrients. 2020;**12**(1):194

[15] Hayward C, Killen JD, Kraemer. T. H. C., C. B.Predictors of panic attacks

in adolescents. Journal of the American Academy of Child & Adolescent Psychiatry. 2000;**39**(2):207-214

[16] Page MJ et al. The PRISMA 2020 statement: An updated guideline for reporting systematic reviews. International Journal of Surgery. 2021;**88**:105906

[17] Hale GE et al. Review: Physical activity interventions for the mental health and well-being of adolescents - a systematic review. Child Adolesc Ment Health. 2021;**26**(4):357-368

[18] Mogre V et al. Adherence to self-care behaviours and associated barriers in type 2 diabetes patients of low-and middle-income countries: A systematic review protocol. Systematic Reviews. 2017;**6**(1):39

[19] Morris SB. Estimating effect sizes from pretest-posttest-control group designs. Organizational research methods. 2008;**11**(2):364-386

[20] Wan X et al. Estimating the sample mean and standard deviation from the sample size, median, range and/ or interquartile range. BMC Medical Research Methodology. 2014;**14**(1):1-13

[21] Higgins JP et al. Cochrane handbook for systematic reviews of interventions. Chichester: John Wiley & Sons. 2019

[22] Efron B. Nonparametric standard errors and confidence intervals. canadian Journal of Statistics. 1981;**9**(2):139-158

[23] Lakens D. Calculating and reporting effect sizes to facilitate cumulative science: A practical primer for t-tests and ANOVAs. Frontiers in Psychology. 2013;**4**:863

[24] Cohen J. Statistical power analysis for the behavioral sciences. New York: Academic press. 2013

[25] Luna P, Guerrero J, Cejudo J. Improving adolescents subjective well-being, trait emotional intelligence and social anxiety through a programme based on the sport education model. International Journal of Environmental Research and Public Health. 2019;**16**(10):1821

[26] Lindwall M, Lindgren EC. The effects of a 6-month exercise intervention programme on physical self-perceptions and social physique anxiety in non-physically active adolescent Swedish girls. Psychology of Sport and Exercise. 2005;**6**(6):643-658

[27] Romero-Perez EM et al. Influence of a physical exercise program in the anxiety and depression in children with obesity. International Journal of Environmental Research and Public Health. 2020;**17**(13):4655

[28] Akko DP et al. The effects of an exercise training on steroid hormones in preadolescent children - a moderator for enhanced cognition? Physiology and Behavior. 2020;**227**:113168

[29] Naderi S et al. The effect of physical exercise on anxiety among the victims of child abuse. Sport Sciences for Health. 2019;**15**(3):519-525

[30] Polis RL et al. Integration of yoga therapy into traditional residential treatment for at risk adolescent females: A community-based approach. Journal of Pediatric and Adolescent Gynecology. 2017;**30**(2):320-321

[31] Smits JA et al. The effects of acute exercise on CO2 challenge reactivity. Journal of Psychiatric Research. 2009;**43**(4):446-454

[32] Broman-Fulks JJ, Storey KM. Evaluation of a brief aerobic exercise intervention for high anxiety

sensitivity. Anxiety, Stress, & Coping. 2008;**21**(2):117-128

[33] Kenis-Coskun Ö et al. The effect of telerehabilitation on quality of life, anxiety, and depression in children with cystic fibrosis and caregivers: A single-blind randomized trial. Pediatric Pulmonology. 2022;**57**(5):1262-1271

[34] Mücke M et al. The influence of an acute exercise bout on adolescents' stress reactivity, interference control, and brain oxygenation under stress. Frontiers in Psychology. 2020;**11**:3091

[35] Wemmie JA. Neurobiology of panic and pH chemosensation in the brain. Dialogues in Clinical Neuroscience. 2022;**13**:475-483

[36] Coryell MW et al. Targeting ASIC1a reduces innate fear and alters neuronal activity in the fear circuit. Biological Psychiatry. 2007;**62**(10):1140-1148

[37] Wemmie JA et al. Acid-sensing ion channel 1 is localized in brain regions with high synaptic density and contributes to fear conditioning. Journal of Neuroscience. 2003;**23**(13):5496-5502

[38] Papp LA et al. Respiratory psychophysiology of panic disorder: Three respiratory challenges in 98 subjects. American Journal of Psychiatry. 1997;**154**(11):1557-1565

[39] Griez E, van Den Hout MA. CO2 inhalation in the treatment of panic attacks. Behaviour Research and Therapy. 1986;**24**(2):145-150

[40] Stewart PA. Independent and dependent variables of acid-base control. Respiration Physiology. 1978;**33**(1):9-26

[41] Maddock RJ et al. Elevated brain lactate responses to neural activation in panic disorder: A dynamic 1H-MRS study. Molecular Psychiatry. 2009;**14**(5):537-545

[42] Sheikh JI et al. Aging and panic disorder: Phenomenology, comorbidity, and risk factors. The American Journal of Geriatric Psychiatry. 2004;**12**(1):102-109

[43] Elkins RM, Pincus DB, Comer JS. A psychometric evaluation of the panic disorder severity scale for children and adolescents. Psychological Assessment. 2014;**26**(2):609

[44] Riske L et al. Lactate in the brain: An update on its relevance to brain energy, neurons, glia and panic disorder. Therapeutic advances in psychopharmacology. 2017;**7**(2):85-89

[45] Martinsen EW et al. Tolerance to intensive exercise and high levels of lactate in panic disorder. Journal of Anxiety Disorders. 1998;**12**(4):333-342

[46] Hiscock DJ et al. Muscle activation, blood lactate, and perceived exertion responses to changing resistance training programming variables. European Journal of Sport Science. 2016;**16**(5):536-544

[47] Teixeira e Seabra AF et al. Age and sex differences in physical activity of Portuguese adolescents. Medicine and Science in Sports and Exercise. 2008;**40**(1):65-70

[48] Courtney JB et al. Autonomous motivation and action planning are longitudinally associated with physical activity during adolescence and early adulthood. Psychology of Sport and Exercise. 2021;**56**:101974

Chapter 7

Evidence-Based Pharmacotherapies for Panic Disorder

Seth Davin Norrholm

Abstract

This chapter presents a review of the primary psychopharmacological interventions for panic disorder and the empirically derived evidence supporting their continued use. Key factors such as dosing, contraindications, safety, tolerability, and polypharmacy are discussed. The chapter will include a currently supported tier structure for pharmacological treatment planning as well as means for how best to tailor regimens to specific patient needs. Comorbidities and practical applications are addressed as well. Lastly, the chapter closes with some emerging pharmacotherapies that show promise but for which empirical evidence supporting their use remains in its infancy.

Keywords: anxiety, pharmacology, antidepressants, benzodiazepines, treatment planning

1. Introduction

1.1 Panic disorder

In large part because this current text has an overall focus on panic disorder, a review of the signs and symptoms of the clinical presentation of panic disorder will not be provided here (please refer to relevant chapters in this book). Rather, the salient features of panic that represent potential pharmacological treatment targets will be highlighted as this chapter proceeds to review drug treatments for this disorder and its subtypes, common comorbidities, and disability. Panic disorder, per DSM-5 criteria, consists of recurrent panic attacks accompanied by at least a 1-month period in which one of the following occurs: (1) persistent concern about having additional attacks or their consequences, or (2) a significant maladaptive change in behavior due to the attacks [1]. Many panic patients display significant fear and avoidance of places and situations in which a panic attack has previously occurred or may occur in the future [termed agoraphobia]. As has been reviewed in several places throughout this text, panic disorder is common (approximately 3.8% prevalence per Western surveys) [2–4], often chronic, and can have a substantial effect on patient level of function and quality of life [5]. In fact, an estimated 15–20% of panic patients treated pharmacologically with leading effective drugs such as tricyclic antidepressants (TCAs), serotonin selective reuptake inhibitors (SSRIs), or benzodiazepines still meet for panic diagnostic criteria or have experienced symptom relapse as measured 6–12 months after treatment [6]. For these reasons, there continues to be compelling rationale for pursuing more effective treatments for this debilitating disorder.

At the time of clinical intake and initial symptom considerations, therapists should be mindful of other existing conditions that may include the presence of panic attacks or panic-like manifestations but are not true panic attacks in the DSM-5 diagnostic sense. Panic-like attacks, and more generalized anxiety, can accompany clinical presentations of depression, bipolar disorder, and substance use or substance withdrawal [1]. In addition, panic- and anxiety-like reactions can be initiated by exposure to stressors and cues related to tangible, "real-life" situations such as occupational, academic, interpersonal, or social difficulties and obstacles; these events would not be considered panic attacks in the diagnostic sense as: (1) they do not occur spontaneously, (2) may be better accounted for by situational aspects or presence of another disorder, or (3) can be considered reasonably predictable or provoked [1].

Panic attacks themselves, by nature, are foundationally physiological and largely driven by a surging activation of the autonomic nervous system (ANS) and, as such, proceed with about a 10-minute or less duration that coincides with arousing activation of the sympathetic division of the ANS followed by subsequent recruitment of the calming parasympathetic division of the ANS. It is this physiological aspect of panic attacks that is highly responsive to acute drug treatments such as a benzodiazepine. Of note, it is also this physiological aspect that leads many panic sufferers to seek primary care providers or urgent/emergent care for acute treatment [7]. The principally psychological elements of concern and worry about future attacks or their consequences, including avoidance of contexts or cues in which an attack may occur, are targeted by psychotherapeutic approaches such as cognitive behavioral therapy. That is not to say that pharmacological solutions cannot influence the clinical impact of psychological interventions [8]. This will be discussed in further detail later in this chapter.

2. Current pharmacological treatment practices for panic disorder

It has been well established that the most effective treatments for panic disorder include psychotherapies that capitalize on cognitive-behavioral methodologies [9]. That being said, it is also well known in psychiatry that pharmacological interventions, whether in tandem with psychotherapy or as a monotherapy, can provide these patients and clients with clinical benefits as well [10]. The heterogeneity of panic disorder, with possible variations in etiology, symptom profile, and underlying neural mechanisms, has resulted in a wide-ranging pharmacological treatment approach spanning multiple drug classes and several putative central nervous system targets and mechanisms of action [11–13]. In general, pharmacotherapies for panic disorder can be classified into first-, second-, and third-line agents with other drug classes often recruited for refractory cases (**Figure 1**). Not surprisingly, first-line treatments include the selective serotonin reuptake inhibitors (SSRIs) and benzodiazepines [14]. The second-line drug interventions for panic include alternative classes of antidepressants including serotonin/norepinephrine reuptake inhibitors (SNRIs), tricyclic antidepressants, monoamine oxidase (MAO) inhibitors, newer serotonin "multimodal" agents, mirtazapine, and to some extent, some antipsychotics and anticonvulsants [14]. Third-line agents are generally represented by beta blockers, buspirone, and hydroxyzine.

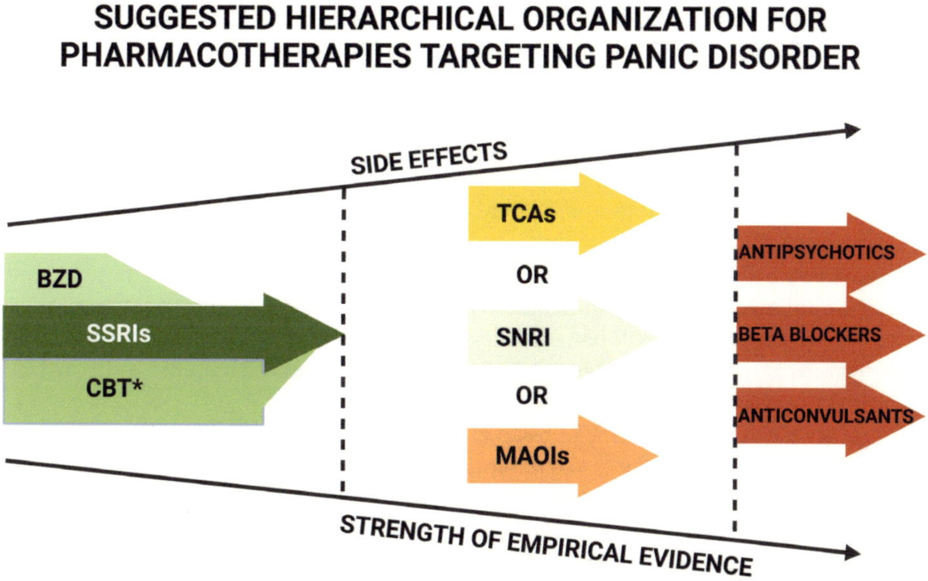

Figure 1.
Schematic illustration of the first-, second-, and third-line pharmacological treatments for panic disorder. Dashed lines indicate an approximation of the division between each drug tier based on the available literature discussed in this chapter. As the drug treatments progress from first- to third-line, there is a general increase in the potential side effects experienced by patients as well as a decrease in the overall empirical data available, either by number of studies performed and/or impact of reported studies. BZD: benzodiazepine; SSRI: serotonin selective reuptake inhibitor; CBT: cognitive behavioral therapy; TCA: tricyclic antidepressant; SNRI: serotonin-norepinephrine reuptake inhibitor; and MAOI: monoamine oxidase inhibitor. Created with BioRender.com.

2.1 First-line pharmacotherapies for panic disorder

2.1.1 Serotonin selective reuptake inhibitors (SSRIs)

Selective serotonin reuptake inhibitors (SSRIs) are a safe and effective pharmacological choice for the treatment of a wide range of mood and anxiety disorders with a large body of empirical evidence supporting their administration [15]; this indication is present for treating panic disorder as well [16–19]. A recent systematic review and meta-analysis by Chawla et al. [14] identified SSRIs as most closely associated with high remission and low risk of adverse events when the most common pharmacotherapies for panic were evaluated with sertraline (trade name Zoloft) and escitalopram (trade name Lexapro) showing clearest clinical benefit [14]. Relatedly, a network analysis by Du et al. [20] of 42 clinical trials encompassing almost 6000 panic disorder patients showed the SSRIs paroxetine, sertraline, fluoxetine, citalopram, and escitalopram to be more efficacious than placebo with the latter drug displaying the most robust efficacy [20].

2.1.2 Benzodiazepines

It is clear from the available empirical literature and clinical guidelines that benzodiazepines are effective in treating many signs and symptoms of panic disorders [16, 21–23] which as described above can include several physiological, stressor- and fear-related features (e.g., tachycardia, rapid breathing, increased perspiration, acute sense of dread, dizziness). In addition, there is effectiveness and safety data supporting the concurrent prescription of benzodiazepines and an antidepressant such as those already mentioned [23]. This may be particularly important during the initial stages of SSRI administration during which time there can be slow onset of SSRI-related benefits and acute increase in panic symptoms [6]. What is not so clear even after decades of research and clinical practice is: (1) the duration for which to prescribe benzodiazepines both short- and long-term, (2) the optimal dosages to use for the available short- and long-acting benzodiazepines, (3) whether or not chronic regimens or as-needed [PRN] indications are more beneficial as compared to the other, (4) the degree to which benzodiazepines may exceed antidepressants for treating panic disorder, or (5) the hierarchical structure for benzodiazepines as organized by clinical benefits [21] .

There is a degree of hesitancy in psychiatry to use benzodiazepines with some patients. This is primarily due to the potential for these drugs to be misused as a result of inherent factors a such as tolerance, dependence, and withdrawal (with its associated potential for rebound effects and symptom relapse). Additionally, there are significant adverse effects to be wary of as clinicians, including but not limited to, sedation, increased risk of falling, impaired memory, and cognitive slowing [17, 22, 24]. As a result, it is important for providers to consider panic disorder patients on a case-by-case basis when selecting antidepressants, benzodiazepines, or a combination of these.

As with many anxiety disorders, panic disorder is associated with incomplete remission and relapse even with first-line pharmacotherapies [14] [and possibly, concomitant psychotherapies]. As such, it is important for treating clinicians to generate a treatment algorithm that accounts for lack of remission, comorbidity, and combined treatment approaches. With regard to transitioning from first-line pharmacological options to a second-line agent, there are some suggestions for how to do so in the available literature. According to Ziffra [16], there are two potential strategies for changing the treatment of a panic patient who has been prescribed monotherapy with an SSRI for a reasonable amount of time with no significant change in symptoms. The first option is to add a second medication to the current SSRI such as a benzodiazepine or another antidepressant. The second alternative is to move to the second-line possibilities, most notably if the patient had little to no improvement with the SSRI alone or could not tolerate the side effects.

2.2 Second-line pharmacotherapies for panic disorder

2.2.1 Serotonin-norepinephrine reuptake inhibitors (SNRIs)

As of this writing, the only FDA-approved serotonin-norepinephrine reuptake inhibitor (SNRI) approved for panic disorder treatment is venlafaxine (trade name Effexor) [25–27]. A number of studies published in the mid-2000s identified superiority of venlafaxine over placebo in reducing panic symptoms in randomized, placebo-controlled, double-blind studies [25, 27–30]. That being said, additional drugs in this class have FDA-approval for treatment of major depressive disorder (MDD) including desvenlafaxine (trade name Pristiq) and duloxetine (trade name Cymbalta) [16]. In addition, despite not having FDA approvals for use with panic disorder patients, there is some open-label evidence available that supports prescribing duloxetine for this clinical population [31] as well as FDA approval for this drug for treating generalized anxiety disorder (GAD) [16].

2.2.2 Tricyclic antidepressants (TCAs)

There is some debate in the field as to whether or not to consider the older tricyclic antidepressants (TCAs) as first- or second-line treatments for panic disorder. In short, the reported efficacy of these drugs, as compared to the SSRIs for example, suggests that they should be treated as first-line agents. However, the side effect profile (e.g., sedation, anticholinergic and cardiac adverse possibilities, weight gain) and potential drug interactions, including with benzodiazepines [14], associated with TCAs provide support for a secondary role within the pharmacological armamentarium available for panic disorder [32].

2.2.3 Monoamine oxidase inhibitors (MAOIs)

While widely considered to be an older antidepressant pharmacotherapy, monoamine oxidase inhibitors (MAOIs; e.g., phenelzine, trade name Nardil) can be considered second- [or possibly third-line] treatments for panic disorder treatment as they have similar side effect concerns and potential medical interactions as TCAs [18]. These potential adverse effects include the need for a low tyramine diet and hypertension monitoring as examples [33]. Yet, there remains strong provider support for keeping this class of drugs as a viable option despite the possible patient adjustments they may require.

2.2.4 "Multimodal" serotonin agents

There are also newer antidepressant drugs that, similar to SSRIs, are FDA-approved for the treatment of MDD and inhibit the reuptake of synaptic serotonin, namely, vilazodone (trade name Viibryd) and vortioxetine (trade names Trintellix/Brintellix). In addition to acting as serotonin reuptake inhibitors, these drugs act at several other classes of serotonin receptors [34] (vortioxetine) including as an agonist at 5-HT1a receptors (vilazodone) [35]. Empirical evidence suggests that these newer antidepressants may be effective for the treatment of panic disorder because of their shared similarity with SSRIs and their enhanced pharmacological profile [36–39].

2.2.5 Mirtazepine

Mirtazapine is one drug for which there is some evidence for use with panic disorder [40] but the available literature is small and, similar to other drugs within this second-line, there are possible adverse effects such as sedation and weight gain to consider [41]. It should be noted here that most of the support for mirtazapine comes from work done over a decade ago and there has been little advancement in recent years.

2.2.6 Anticonvulsants

Clinical evidence supporting the use of anticonvulsants with panic disorder patients comes from the success of these drugs in treating bipolar disorder [42–45] and, as such, the list of candidate agents includes topiramate, lamotrigine, carbamazepine, oxcarbazepine, valproic acid, gabapentin, and pregabalin. The most compelling empirical and clinical arguments, albeit somewhat limited, for using anticonvulsants with panic disorder are available for the latter three drugs. Valproic acid [trade name Depakote] acts at the primary inhibitory GABAergic transmitter systems in the brain and, as such, may help attenuate panic symptoms. Valproic acid is used for mood stabilization in bipolar disorder including in the presence of co-morbid panic [45]. However, as with most of its prescribing practices, valproic acid pharmacotherapy requires close monitoring due to its side effects profile and potential to alter some metabolic functions [46]. The evidence for prescribing gabapentin and pregabalin for panic disorder is scant and consists primarily of a few individual patient cases and open-label trials [47–49]. In addition, there is no FDA approval for the use of these two drugs in anxiety disorders nor is there enough evidence to formulate a treatment algorithm encompassing dosage level, frequency of dosage, or single versus in-tandem, multidrug administration [16]. As such, gabapentin and pregabalin are listed here by drug classification only and not in line with a treatment algorithm. There is simply insufficient evidence to describe them as even a third-line option.

2.3 Third-line pharmacotherapies for panic disorder

2.3.1 Antipsychotics

Selecting an antipsychotic pharmacotherapy for panic disorder likely represents an option when all others have been exhausted. In terms of first-generation (e.g., haloperidol, trade name Haldol) or second-generation antipsychotics (e.g., quetiapine, trade name Seroquel), there exists no available literature supporting their use or very little empirical evidence, respectively, with regard to with panic disorder [50]. In fact, a systematic review of the use of second-generation antipsychotics for anxiety disorders as a whole yielded no positive results [51]. As of this writing, there is a glimmer of support for prescribing quetiapine for GAD but nothing to suggest a use for panic disorder [16]. Lastly and understandably so, there exists no FDA approval for treating panic disorder with antipsychotics [16, 50].

2.3.2 Beta blockers

As mentioned in the Introduction, panic attacks by nature have a psychophysiological component to them as they mirror activation of the sympathetic nervous system complete with tachycardia and perception of impending threat. For this reason, there is compelling rationale to use beta blockers to stem many of these physiological effects; an approach consistent with the acute use of beta blockers to prevent hyper-arousals stemming from performance-based tasks like public speaking [52]. However, the potential clinical advantage of using beta blockers to prevent panic-related somatic manifestations and distress is surprisingly weak [11, 53] and thus relegates these drugs to the third-line tier at best.

2.3.3 Buspirone

The 5-HT1a partial agonist, buspirone, can be considered a third-line treatment option for panic disorder but that standing is somewhat tenuous given that: (1) there is only a small body of literature supporting its use here, (2) the best evidence appears to be its administration with a concomitant antidepressant, (3) the available literature reveals notable adverse effects and a high dropout rate [14], and (4) its FDA approval for treatment of anxiety disorders is limited to generalized anxiety disorder (GAD) [16, 54].

2.3.4 Hydroxyzine

An antihistamine with sedative properties, there is some small support of its use for anxiety, including panic disorder [55]. Despite having FDA approval for use with GAD, empirical evidence of hydroxyzine effectiveness for GAD is mixed [56–58]. Thus, one can consider administering hydroxyzine for panic disorder symptoms as a tertiary strategy [16].

3. Treatment planning

3.1 Assessment of comorbidities

A critical step in treatment planning for clients with possible panic disorder is the assessment of other psychological comorbidities, general medical conditions, or substance related elevations in arousal (e.g., caffeine, cannabis) that may mimic signs and symptoms of panic. With regard to the first factor, it is generally well established that anxiety disorders tend to cluster with one another from a symptomatologic and etiological standpoint [59]. As such, it is imperative for the treating clinician to address any barriers to treatment or exacerbation of symptoms presented by comorbidity. Common psychiatric comorbidities [and potential risk factors for developing panic disorder] include, but are not limited to, depression, substance use, disordered personality, and other anxiety disorders [16, 60–63]. In consideration of the second factor, client and therapist should rule out any potential conditions that could be subjectively reported as panic attacks, including but not limited to, hyperthyroidism, epilepsy, hypoglycemia, cardiac issues, asthma or respiratory ailments, or dizziness/vertigo [16]. Regarding substance intake, clinicians should perform some type of timeline follow-back query to assess the client's use of food, drink, consumables, or recreational drugs known to increase psychophysiological arousal. Relatedly, assessment of substance-induced anxiety disorder should occur as well.

3.2 Course of treatment: how much of which drug and for how long?

A critical question for which clinicians are still seeking answers is the type and duration of pharmacological interventions for panic disorder. There is still considerable debate regarding several key questions including, but not limited to: (1) for how long should patients take anti-panic medications to best ensure relapse is minimal and gains are maintained, (2) if medications are to be taken long-term, should maintenance doses be reduced or held at short-term therapeutic levels, (3) of the medications reviewed here, are there some that outperform others when length of treatment becomes the issue, (4) what are the persistent, or newly emerging, side effects of which to be wary, and (5) are there identifiable clinical or individual predictors of short- and long-term treatment outcome and relapse suppression? There have been a small number of clinical studies that have sought to answer these questions.

Two randomized trials conducted in the last decade investigated the long-term efficacy of two supported pharmacotherapies for panic disorder, SSRIs and clonazepam, administered in tandem with another type of treatment (CBT) or as compared to an alternative drug regimen [paroxetine], respectively. Nardi et al. [64] compared long-term (34 months) treatment with paroxetine or clonazepam in a study extended from an ongoing short-term investigation of the medications [64, 65]. In the earlier short-term study, both paroxetine and clonazepam displayed similar reductions in the patient-reported number of panic attacks and in overall level of anxiety as assessed with Hamilton Anxiety and Clinical Global Impression-Severity scores [65]. Patients reported a faster onset of drug effects and fewer adverse events with clonazepam as compared to paroxetine in the short-term. These effects on panic attack reduction and diminished anxiety held true for the long-term extension as did the fewer number of adverse events regarding clonazepam over paroxetine. Not surprisingly, the adverse events reported with clonazepam use were drowsiness and fatigue as well as impairments in memory and concentration while with long-term paroxetine, patients reported change in appetite and weight gain as well as diarrhea, constipation, and dry mouth.

A second long-term study of note directly compared the parallel combination of CBT and SSRIs with each treatment arm alone [66]. When assed over a 1-year treatment period, CBT + SSRI, CBT alone, and SSRI alone all resulted in a significant reduction in panic attack frequency. Of note, patients who received CBT alone reported a slower decline in panic attacks over time and more spontaneous panic attacks during the past year. The authors of this long-term study also highlight that patient symptoms improved at a faster rate with combined CBT and SSRIs particularly in those patients with co-occurring agoraphobia [66]. As will be discussed in the next section, there is certainly evidence for drug monotherapies for panic disorder but the most significant clinical gains may arise from the combination of pharmacotherapy with psychotherapy. In addition, most of the emerging data from this area suggest maintenance therapy of up to a year or more after an initial course of pharmacological treatment and symptom reduction [6].

3.3 Co-administration of pharmacotherapies with psychotherapy

The primary focus of this chapter is on the use of pharmacological agents to treat the signs and symptoms of panic disorder. However, this chapter would be incomplete if it did not highlight the importance of psychotherapy—namely cognitive behavioral therapy (CBT) for the effective treatment of panic disorder. The most effective interventions for anxiety disorders are CBT-based (for review see Otto and Deveney [67]) and, as such, therapists should seek out ways in which CBT and pharmacotherapy can mutually benefit one another [23, 67]. In addition, as alluded to earlier in this chapter, benzodiazepines are intended for short-term usage for management of panic symptoms and should be tapered when clinically indicated. This weaning can produce a withdrawal process that can acutely exacerbate panic and it is often recommended that a program such as Panic Control Treatment for Benzodiazepine (BZ) discontinuation be incorporated into treatment plans [68–72].

4. Future directions and exploratory pharmacotherapies

In order to address the shortcomings of the currently available pharmacotherapies for panic disorder, there has been a renewed interest in psychiatry in exploring additional alternative drug therapies. The search for new and innovative medications, for mood and anxiety disorders more broadly, has included psychedelics such as 3,4-methylenedioxymethamphetamine (MDMA), increasingly legal and available cannabinoids, orexinergic compounds, glutamatergic agents (e.g., D-Cycloserine, esketamine), and anesthetics (e.g., Xenon gas). As of this writing, scant empirical evidence exists to support the use of MDMA nor cannabinoids for panic disorder and there are, in fact, studies that suggest that the use of the latter class of drugs could be problematic [73, 74]. There are, as will be seen below, encouraging emerging findings supporting the use of compounds that act on orexin systems as well as the anesthetic, xenon.

4.1 Orexinergic pathways as a drug target for treating panic disorder

The orexin system is of particular interest as a pharmacological target for treating panic disorder due to the putative role of this neuropeptide in the underlying pathophysiology of panic including its regulatory functions related to chemo-, cardio-, and behavioral responses to fluctuations in CO2 and H+ [13, 75]. For example, activity within orexinergic hypothalamic neurons and along brainstem cardiorespiratory pathways is increased by CO2 or NaLac challenge [76, 77]. In addition, expression of orexin-1 receptors is rich in areas shown to mediate defensive, emotional, arousal and panic-like behaviors such as the noradrenergic locus coeruleus, serotonergic raphe nucleus, brainstem cardiorespiratory maintenance nuclei, the extended limbic system, and the periaqueductal gray [78, 79]. Consistent with this expression of orexin-1 receptors, selective antagonists can block panic behaviors and cardiovascular responses induced by CO2 challenge, at least when administered directly into the raphe [80].

A recent systematic review by Caldirola et al. [13] examined the empirical, translational evidence supporting the use of orexin receptor antagonists to treat panic disorder. The work reviewed by this group assessed compounds at iterative stages of drug development including preclinical animal studies and Phase I trials with psychiatrically healthy human participants. In the preclinical animal studies, investigators employed commonly used paradigms to produce panic-like behaviors in rodents including external (e.g., cage exchange between housed animal groups) and internal (e.g., sodium lactate, NaLac, injection or 20% CO2 inhalation) stressors. Systematic review by Caldirola's team identified three orexin-1 receptor selective antagonists, compound 56, JNJ-54717793, and JNJ-61393215, that displayed an ability to block panic behaviors and cardiovascular responses induced by the aforementioned paradigms. Notably, there were some differences in effectiveness between tested compounds and as compared to benzodiazepine controls but each appeared to be effective without sedative effects or significant effects on sleep-wake cycles [13, 81–83]. Lastly, selective orexin-2 receptor antagonists did not show any significant capacity to block panic-related behaviors and responses.

The animal studies alluded to above were then subsequently followed by Phase I human trials with healthy participants. For example, Salvadore et al. [83] found that the selective orexin-1 receptor selective antagonist, JNJ-61393215, possessed a good tolerability and safety profile, showed no drowsiness or cardiovascular effects, and significantly reduced panic symptoms induced by a 35% CO2 inhalation challenge when assessed in healthy males. Complementary work by Kaufmann et al. [84] suggested that the selective orexin-1 receptor antagonist, ACT-539313, was generally safe and well tolerated with some reports of somnolence. Yet, the anxiolytic potential of this compound requires further exploration as early evidence suggests it may reduce anxiety associated with a 7.5% CO2 challenge but not necessarily test-elicited panic symptoms [84]. It is clear as of this writing that there remains much translational work to be done before the orexin-1 receptor antagonist class of drugs can be considered for panic disorder treatment.

4.2 Glutamatergic pathways as a drug target for treating panic disorder

In terms of glutamatergic agents acting as potential anti-panic medications, there is compelling data from the treatment of other anxiety and mood disorders that warrant further investigation. The antibiotic and partial NMDA receptor agonist, D-Cylcoserine (DCS), for example, has a recent history of potential use as a cognitive enhancer that may facilitate cognitive behavioral therapies (CBTs) for anxiety disorders such as specific phobias under specific therapeutic conditions [85]. The use of DCS as an adjunctive treatment for panic-related CBT was recently examined by Reinecke et al. [86] who showed that while DCS reduced bias for threatening faces and associated amygdala activity, it did not differ from placebo on clinical measures of panic-related signs and symptoms [86].

As of this writing, the anti-panic properties of esketamine have not been fully explored and the strongest data available support the use of ketamines as a rapid-onset pharmacotherapy for treatment resistant depression [87], but not yet for anxiety disorders.

The inhalation of the anesthetic, xenon, has been studied recently as a potential pharmacotherapy for panic disorder [88], in part because of the gas' ability to decrease excitatory neurotransmission via interactions at glutamatergic NMDA and AMPA, serotonergic 5HT-3, and cholinergic nicotinic receptors [11, 89]. Dobrovolsky et al. [88] administered 6–7 inhalations of xenon at a sub-anesthetic dose for 2.4–4 minutes to a study sample consisting of panic disorder patients with and without psychiatric comorbidity. Symptom ratings, as measured by the Hospital Anxiety and Depression Scale and Zung Self-rating, global impression ratings, and frequency of panic attackers were all reduced following the xenon inhalations, with many patients reporting benefits after only 3 treatments. The authors reported xenon to be well tolerated, however, provided no putative mechanism of action. Continuing work with greater rigor and replicability than the existing studies should provide further insight into this unconventional, yet cautiously promising, delivery of panic disorder treatment.

5. Conclusions

The available empirical and clinical evidence suggests that first-line pharmacotherapies for panic disorder include selective serotonin reuptake inhibitors (SSRIs) and benzodiazepines with the former best accompanied by cognitive behavioral therapy (CBT) and the latter used for short-term management of panic symptoms (**Figure 1**). In refractory cases, there are second- and third-line pharmacological agents available, however, their use has mixed results and support, possesses less clear treatment regimens and algorithms, and comes with increasing possibility of side effects and adverse interactions. Emerging clinical data from the study of mood disorders, including MDD, suggest that serotonin multimodal drugs and faster acting medications like esketamine may show promise moving forward. One can imagine that the next decade of drug development in the area of panic disorder will represent an amalgam of evidence gleaned from the pharmacological treatment of disorders with which panic is co-morbid, serendipitous findings from the clinic that continue to shed light on new innovations, and a maintenance of the psycho/pharmacotherapy regimen that has shown efficacy for the better part of the past 25 years.

Conflict of interest

The author declares no conflict of interest.

Author details

Seth Davin Norrholm[1,2]

1 Department of Psychiatry and Behavioral Neurosciences, Wayne State University School of Medicine, Detroit, Michigan, USA

2 Department of Behavioral Sciences and Leadership, United States Air Force Academy, Colorado, USA

*Address all correspondence to: snorrholm@wayne.edu

References

[1] American Psychiatric Association. Diagnostic and Statistical Manual of Mental Disorders, Fifth Edition, DSM-5. Arlington, VA: American Psychiatric Association; 2013

[2] Kessler RC, Petukhova M, Sampson NA, Zaslavsky AM, Wittchen HU. Twelve-month and lifetime prevalence and lifetime morbid risk of anxiety and mood disorders in the United States. International Journal of Methods in Psychiatric Research. 2012;**21**(3):169-184

[3] de Jonge P, Roest AM, Lim CC, Florescu SE, Bromet EJ, Stein DJ, et al. Cross-national epidemiology of panic disorder and panic attacks in the world mental health surveys. Depression and Anxiety. 2016;**33**(12):1155-1177

[4] Skapinakis P, Lewis G, Davies S, Brugha T, Prince M, Singleton N. Panic disorder and subthreshold panic in the UK general population: Epidemiology, comorbidity and functional limitation. European Psychiatry. 2011;**26**(6):354-362

[5] Batelaan N, Smit F, de Graaf R, van Balkom A, Vollebergh W, Beekman A. Economic costs of full-blown and subthreshold panic disorder. Journal of Affective Disorders. 2007;**104**(1-3):127-136

[6] Batelaan NM, Van Balkom AJ, Stein DJ. Evidence-based pharmacotherapy of panic disorder: An update. The International Journal of Neuropsychopharmacology. 2012;**15**(3):403-415

[7] Katerndahl DA, Realini JP. Where do panic attack sufferers seek care? The Journal of Family Practice. 1995;**40**(3):237-243

[8] Marazziti D, Carlini M, Dell'Osso L. Treatment strategies of obsessive-compulsive disorder and panic disorder/agoraphobia. Current Topics in Medicinal Chemistry. 2012;**12**(4):238-253

[9] Aaronson CJ, Shear MK, Goetz RR, Allen LB, Barlow DH, White KS, et al. Predictors and time course of response among panic disorder patients treated with cognitive-behavioral therapy. The Journal of Clinical Psychiatry. 2008;**69**(3):418-424

[10] Roy-Byrne PP, Craske MG, Stein MB. Panic disorder. Lancet. 2006;**368**(9540):1023-1032

[11] Caldirola D, Alciati A, Riva A, Perna G. Are there advances in pharmacotherapy for panic disorder? A systematic review of the past five years. Expert Opinion on Pharmacotherapy. 2018;**19**(12):1357-1368

[12] Caldirola D, Alciati A, Dacco S, Micieli W, Perna G. Relapse prevention in panic disorder with pharmacotherapy: Where are we now? Expert Opinion on Pharmacotherapy. 2020;**21**(14):1699-1711

[13] Caldirola D, Alciati A, Cuniberti F, Perna G. Experimental drugs for panic disorder: An updated systematic review. Journal of Experimental Pharmacology. 2021;**13**:441-459

[14] Chawla N, Anothaisintawee T, Charoenrungrueangchai K, Thaipisuttikul P, McKay GJ, Attia J, et al. Drug treatment for panic disorder with or without agoraphobia: Systematic review and network meta-analysis of randomised controlled trials. BMJ. 2022;**376**:e066084

[15] Vaswani M, Linda FK, Ramesh S. Role of selective serotonin reuptake

inhibitors in psychiatric disorders: A comprehensive review. Progress in Neuro-Psychopharmacology & Biological Psychiatry. 2003;**27**(1):85-102

[16] Ziffra M. Panic disorder: A review of treatment options. Annals of Clinical Psychiatry. 2021;**33**(2):124-133

[17] Bighelli I, Castellazzi M, Cipriani A, Girlanda F, Guaiana G, Koesters M, et al. Antidepressants versus placebo for panic disorder in adults. Cochrane Database of Systematic Reviews. 2018;**4**:CD010676

[18] Bakker A, van Balkom AJ, Spinhoven P. SSRIs vs. TCAs in the treatment of panic disorder: A meta-analysis. Acta Psychiatrica Scandinavica. 2002;**106**(3):163-167

[19] Boyer W. Serotonin uptake inhibitors are superior to imipramine and alprazolam in alleviating panic attacks: A meta-analysis. International Clinical Psychopharmacology. 1995;**10**(1):45-49

[20] Du Y, Du B, Diao Y, Yin Z, Li J, Shu Y, et al. Comparative efficacy and acceptability of antidepressants and benzodiazepines for the treatment of panic disorder: A systematic review and network meta-analysis. Asian Journal of Psychiatry. 2021;**60**:102664

[21] Bighelli I, Trespidi C, Castellazzi M, Cipriani A, Furukawa TA, Girlanda F, et al. Antidepressants and benzodiazepines for panic disorder in adults. Cochrane Database of Systematic Reviews. 2016;**9**:CD011567

[22] Breilmann J, Girlanda F, Guaiana G, Barbui C, Cipriani A, Castellazzi M, et al. Benzodiazepines versus placebo for panic disorder in adults. Cochrane Database of Systematic Reviews. 2019;**3**:CD010677

[23] Workgroup on Panic Disorder APA. Practice guideline for the treatment of patients with panic disorder. American Journal of Psychiatry. 1998;**155**:1-34

[24] Bruce SE, Vasile RG, Goisman RM, Salzman C, Spencer M, Machan JT, et al. Are benzodiazepines still the medication of choice for patients with panic disorder with or without agoraphobia? The American Journal of Psychiatry. 2003;**160**(8):1432-1438

[25] Pollack M, Mangano R, Entsuah R, Tzanis E, Simon NM, Zhang Y. A randomized controlled trial of venlafaxine ER and paroxetine in the treatment of outpatients with panic disorder. Psychopharmacology. 2007;**194**(2): 233-242

[26] Ferguson JM, Khan A, Mangano R, Entsuah R, Tzanis E. Relapse prevention of panic disorder in adult outpatient responders to treatment with venlafaxine extended release. The Journal of Clinical Psychiatry. 2007;**68**(1):58-68

[27] Bradwejn J, Ahokas A, Stein DJ, Salinas E, Emilien G, Whitaker T. Venlafaxine extended-release capsules in panic disorder: Flexible-dose, double-blind, placebo-controlled study. The British Journal of Psychiatry. 2005;**187**:352-359

[28] Liebowitz MR, Asnis G, Mangano R, Tzanis E. A double-blind, placebo-controlled, parallel-group, flexible-dose study of venlafaxine extended release capsules in adult outpatients with panic disorder. The Journal of Clinical Psychiatry. 2009;**70**(4):550-561

[29] Pollack MH, Lepola U, Koponen H, Simon NM, Worthington JJ, Emilien G, et al. A double-blind study of the efficacy of venlafaxine extended-release, paroxetine, and placebo in the treatment of panic disorder. Depression and Anxiety. 2007;**24**(1):1-14

[30] Kjernisted K, McIntosh D. Venlafaxine extended release (XR) in the treatment of panic disorder. Therapeutics and Clinical Risk Management. 2007;**3**(1):59-69

[31] Simon NM, Kaufman RE, Hoge EA, Worthington JJ, Herlands NN, Owens ME, et al. Open-label support for duloxetine for the treatment of panic disorder. CNS Neuroscience & Therapeutics. 2009;**15**(1):19-23

[32] Bandelow B, Michaelis S, Wedekind D. Treatment of anxiety disorders. Dialogues in Clinical Neuroscience. 2017;**19**(2):93-107

[33] Stahl SM, Felker A. Monoamine oxidase inhibitors: A modern guide to an unrequited class of antidepressants. CNS Spectrums. 2008;**13**(10):855-870

[34] Gonda X, Sharma SR, Tarazi FI. Vortioxetine: A novel antidepressant for the treatment of major depressive disorder. Expert Opinion on Drug Discovery. 2019;**14**(1):81-89

[35] Sahli ZT, Banerjee P, Tarazi FI. The preclinical and clinical effects of Vilazodone for the treatment of major depressive disorder. Expert Opinion on Drug Discovery. 2016;**11**(5):515-523

[36] Stuivenga M, Giltay EJ, Cools O, Roosens L, Neels H, Sabbe B. Evaluation of vilazodone for the treatment of depressive and anxiety disorders. Expert Opinion on Pharmacotherapy. 2019;**20**(3):251-260

[37] Sowa-Kucma M, Panczyszyn-Trzewik P, Misztak P, Jaeschke RR, Sendek K, Styczen K, et al. Vortioxetine: A review of the pharmacology and clinical profile of the novel antidepressant. Pharmacological Reports. 2017;**69**(4):595-601

[38] Pae CU, Wang SM, Han C, Lee SJ, Patkar AA, Masand PS, et al. Vortioxetine, a multimodal antidepressant for generalized anxiety disorder: A systematic review and meta-analysis. Journal of Psychiatric Research. 2015;**64**:88-98

[39] Shah A, Northcutt J. An open-label, flexible dose adaptive study evaluating the efficacy of vortioxetine in subjects with panic disorder. Annals of General Psychiatry. 2018;**17**:19

[40] Carli V, Sarchiapone M, Camardese G, Romano L, DeRisio S. Mirtazapine in the treatment of panic disorder. Archives of General Psychiatry. 2002;**59**(7):661-662

[41] Carpenter LL, Leon Z, Yasmin S, Price LH. Clinical experience with mirtazapine in the treatment of panic disorder. Annals of Clinical Psychiatry. 1999;**11**(2):81-86

[42] Mula M, Pini S, Cassano GB. The role of anticonvulsant drugs in anxiety disorders: A critical review of the evidence. Journal of Clinical Psychopharmacology. 2007;**27**:263-272

[43] Van Ameringen M, Mancini C, Pipe B, Bennett M. Antiepileptic drugs in the treatment of anxiety disorders: Role in therapy. Drugs. 2004;**64**(19):2199-2220

[44] Boutros NN, Ghosh S, Khan A, Bowyer SM, Galloway MP. Anticonvulsant medications for panic disorder: A review and synthesis of the evidence. International Journal of Psychiatry in Clinical Practice. 2014;**18**(1):2-10

[45] Rakofsky JJ, Dunlop BW. Treating nonspecific anxiety and anxiety disorders in patients with bipolar

disorder: A review. The Journal of Clinical Psychiatry. 2011;**72**(1):81-90

[46] Davis R, Peters DH, McTavish D. Valproic acid. A reappraisal of its pharmacological properties and clinical efficacy in epilepsy. Drugs. 1994;**47**(2):332-372

[47] Joos AA, Zeeck A. Gabapentin in somatoform and panic disorder. Journal of Clinical Psychopharmacology. 2013;**33**(1):140-142

[48] Lauria-Horner BA, Pohl RB. Pregabalin: A new anxiolytic. Expert Opinion on Investigational Drugs. 2003;**12**(4):663-672

[49] Montgomery S, Emir B, Haswell H, Prieto R. Long-term treatment of anxiety disorders with pregabalin: A 1 year open-label study of safety and tolerability. Current Medical Research and Opinion. 2013;**29**(10):1223-1230

[50] Perna G, Alessandra A, Raffaele B, Elisa M, Giuseppina D, Paolo C, et al. Is there room for second-generation antipsychotics in the pharmacotherapy of panic disorder? A systematic review based on PRISMA guidelines. International Journal of Molecular Sciences. 2016;**17**(4):551

[51] Depping AM, Komossa K, Kissling W, Leucht S. Second-generation antipsychotics for anxiety disorders. Cochrane Database of Systematic Reviews. 2010;**12**:CD008120

[52] Davidson JR. Pharmacotherapy of social anxiety disorder: What does the evidence tell us? The Journal of Clinical Psychiatry. 2006;**67**(Suppl 12):20-26

[53] Steenen SA, van Wijk AJ, van der Heijden GJ, van Westrhenen R, de Lange J, de Jongh A. Propranolol for the treatment of anxiety disorders: Systematic review and meta-analysis. Journal of Psychopharmacology. 2016;**30**(2):128-139

[54] Imai H, Tajika A, Chen P, Pompoli A, Guaiana G, Castellazzi M, et al. Azapirones versus placebo for panic disorder in adults. Cochrane Database of Systematic Reviews. 2014;**9**:CD010828

[55] Iskandar JW, Griffeth B, Rubio-Cespedes C. Successful treatment with hydroxyzine of acute exacerbation of panic disorder in a healthy man: A case report. Primary Care Companion for CNS Disorders. 2011;**13**(3)

[56] Guaiana G, Barbui C, Cipriani A. Hydroxyzine for generalised anxiety disorder. Cochrane Database of Systematic Reviews. 2010;**12**:CD006815

[57] Llorca PM, Spadone C, Sol O, Danniau A, Bougerol T, Corruble E, et al. Efficacy and safety of hydroxyzine in the treatment of generalized anxiety disorder: A 3-month double-blind study. The Journal of Clinical Psychiatry. 2002;**63**(11):1020-1027

[58] Ferreri M, Hantouche EG. Recent clinical trials of hydroxyzine in generalized anxiety disorder. Acta Psychiatrica Scandinavica. Supplementum. 1998;**393**:102-108

[59] Penninx BW, Pine DS, Holmes EA, Reif A. Anxiety disorders. Lancet. 2021;**397**(10277):914-927

[60] Lecrubier Y. The impact of comorbidity on the treatment of panic disorder. The Journal of Clinical Psychiatry. 1998;**59**(Suppl 8):11-14; discussion 5-6

[61] Marshall JR. Alcohol and substance abuse in panic disorder. The Journal of

Clinical Psychiatry. 1997;**58**(Suppl 2):46-49; discussion 9-50

[62] Zvolensky MJ, Bernstein A, Marshall EC, Feldner MT. Panic attacks, panic disorder, and agoraphobia: Associations with substance use, abuse, and dependence. Current Psychiatry Reports. 2006;**8**(4):279-285

[63] Kessler RC, Chiu WT, Jin R, Ruscio AM, Shear K, Walters EE. The epidemiology of panic attacks, panic disorder, and agoraphobia in the National Comorbidity Survey Replication. Archives of General Psychiatry. 2006;**63**(4):415-424

[64] Nardi AE, Freire RC, Mochcovitch MD, Amrein R, Levitan MN, King AL, et al. A randomized, naturalistic, parallel-group study for the long-term treatment of panic disorder with clonazepam or paroxetine. Journal of Clinical Psychopharmacology. 2012;**32**(1):120-126

[65] Nardi AE, Valenca AM, Freire RC, Amrein R, Sardinha A, Levitan MN, et al. Randomized, open naturalistic, acute treatment of panic disorder with clonazepam or paroxetine. Journal of Clinical Psychopharmacology. 2011;**31**(2):259-261

[66] Van Apeldoorn FJ, Van Hout WJ, Timmerman ME, Mersch PP, den Boer JA. Rate of improvement during and across three treatments for panic disorder with or without agoraphobia: Cognitive behavioral therapy, selective serotonin reuptake inhibitor or both combined. Journal of Affective Disorders. 2013;**150**(2):313-319

[67] Otto MW, Deveney C. Cognitive-behavioral therapy and the treatment of panic disorder: Efficacy and strategies. The Journal of Clinical Psychiatry. 2005;**66**(Suppl 4):28-32

[68] Spiegel DA, Bruce TJ, Gregg SF, Nuzzarello A. Does cognitive behavior therapy assist slow-taper alprazolam discontinuation in panic disorder? The American Journal of Psychiatry. 1994;**151**(6):876-881

[69] Otto MW, Pollack MH, Meltzer-BrodyS, RosenbaumJF. Cognitive-behavioral therapy for benzodiazepine discontinuation in panic disorder patients. Psychopharmacology Bulletin. 1992;**28**(2):123-130

[70] Otto MW, Pollack MH, Sachs GS, Reiter SR, Meltzer-Brody S, Rosenbaum JF. Discontinuation of benzodiazepine treatment: Efficacy of cognitive-behavioral therapy for patients with panic disorder. The American Journal of Psychiatry. 1993;**150**(10):1485-1490

[71] Otto MW, Hong JJ, Safren SA. Benzodiazepine discontinuation difficulties in panic disorder: Conceptual model and outcome for cognitive-behavior therapy. Current Pharmaceutical Design. 2002;**8**(1):75-80

[72] Otto MW, McHugh RK, Simon NM, Farach FJ, Worthington JJ, Pollack MH. Efficacy of CBT for benzodiazepine discontinuation in patients with panic disorder: Further evaluation. Behaviour Research and Therapy. 2010;**48**(8):720-727

[73] Petrowski K, Conrad R. Comparison of cortisol stress response in patients with panic disorder, cannabis-induced panic disorder, and healthy controls. Psychopathology. 2019;**52**(1):26-32

[74] Zvolensky MJ, Bernstein A, Sachs-Ericsson N, Schmidt NB, Buckner JD, Bonn-Miller MO. Lifetime associations between cannabis, use, abuse, and dependence and panic attacks in a representative sample.

Journal of Psychiatric Research. 2006;**40**(6):477-486

[75] Johnson PL, Federici LM, Fitz SD, Renger JJ, Shireman B, Winrow CJ, et al. Orexin 1 and 2 receptor involvement in Co2 -induced panic-associated behavior and autonomic responses. Depression and Anxiety. 2015;**32**(9):671-683

[76] Johnson PL, Fitz SD, Hollis JH, Moratalla R, Lightman SL, Shekhar A, et al. Induction of c-Fos in 'panic/defence'-related brain circuits following brief hypercarbic gas exposure. Journal of Psychopharmacology. 2011;**25**(1):26-36

[77] Johnson PL, Truitt W, Fitz SD, Minick PE, Dietrich A, Sanghani S, et al. A key role for orexin in panic anxiety. Nature Medicine. 2010;**16**(1):111-115

[78] Nattie E, Li A. Respiration and autonomic regulation and orexin. Progress in Brain Research. 2012;**198**:25-46

[79] Johnson PL, Samuels BC, Fitz SD, Federici LM, Hammes N, Early MC, et al. Orexin 1 receptors are a novel target to modulate panic responses and the panic brain network. Physiology & Behavior. 2012;**107**(5):733-742

[80] Johnson PL, Samuels BC, Fitz SD, Lightman SL, Lowry CA, Shekhar A. Activation of the orexin 1 receptor is a critical component of CO2-mediated anxiety and hypertension but not bradycardia. Neuropsychopharmacology. 2012;**37**(8):1911-1922

[81] Bonaventure P, Yun S, Johnson PL, Shekhar A, Fitz SD, Shireman BT, et al. A selective orexin-1 receptor antagonist attenuates stress-induced hyperarousal without hypnotic effects. The Journal of Pharmacology and Experimental Therapeutics. 2015;**352**(3):590-601

[82] Bonaventure P, Dugovic C, Shireman B, Preville C, Yun S, Lord B, et al. Evaluation of JNJ-54717793 a novel brain penetrant selective orexin 1 receptor antagonist in two rat models of panic attack provocation. Frontiers in Pharmacology. 2017;**8**:357

[83] Salvadore G, Bonaventure P, Shekhar A, Johnson PL, Lord B, Shireman BT, et al. Translational evaluation of novel selective orexin-1 receptor antagonist JNJ-61393215 in an experimental model for panic in rodents and humans. Translational Psychiatry. 2020;**10**(1):308

[84] Kaufmann P, Ort M, Golor G, Kornberger R, Dingemanse J. Multiple-dose clinical pharmacology of the selective orexin-1 receptor antagonist ACT-539313. Progress in Neuro-Psychopharmacology & Biological Psychiatry. 2021;**108**:110166

[85] Mataix-Cols D, Fernandez de la Cruz L, Monzani B, Rosenfield D, Andersson E, Perez-Vigil A, et al. D-Cycloserine augmentation of exposure-based cognitive behavior therapy for anxiety, obsessive-compulsive, and posttraumatic stress disorders: A systematic review and meta-analysis of individual participant data. JAMA. Psychiatry. 2017;**74**(5):501-510

[86] Reinecke A, Nickless A, Browning M, Harmer CJ. Neurocognitive processes in d-cycloserine augmented single-session exposure therapy for anxiety: A randomized placebo-controlled trial. Behaviour Research and Therapy. 2020;**129**:103607

[87] Lee EE, Della Selva MP, Liu A, Himelhoch S. Ketamine as a novel treatment for major depressive disorder and bipolar depression: A systematic review and quantitative meta-analysis. General Hospital Psychiatry. 2015;**37**(2):178-184

[88] Dobrovolsky A, Ichim TE, Ma D, Kesari S, Bogin V. Xenon in the treatment of panic disorder: An open label study. Journal of Translational Medicine. 2017;**15**(1):137

[89] Zhou C, Liu J, Chen XD. General anesthesia mediated by effects on ion channels. World Journal of Critical Care Medicine. 2012;**1**(3):80-93